Urothelial Carcinoma: Clinical Diagnosis and Treatment

Urothelial Carcinoma: Clinical Diagnosis and Treatment

Editor

Massimiliano Creta

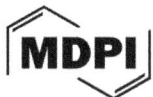

Basel • Beijing • Wuhan • Barcelona • Belgrade • Novi Sad • Cluj • Manchester

Editor
Massimiliano Creta
University of Naples Federico II
Naples, Italy

Editorial Office
MDPI
St. Alban-Anlage 66
4052 Basel, Switzerland

This is a reprint of articles from the Special Issue published online in the open access journal *Journal of Clinical Medicine* (ISSN 2077-0383) (available at: https://www.mdpi.com/journal/jcm/special_issues/Clinical_Urothelial_Carcinoma).

For citation purposes, cite each article independently as indicated on the article page online and as indicated below:

Lastname, A.A.; Lastname, B.B. Article Title. *Journal Name* **Year**, *Volume Number*, Page Range.

ISBN 978-3-0365-8824-7 (Hbk)
ISBN 978-3-0365-8825-4 (PDF)
doi.org/10.3390/books978-3-0365-8825-4

© 2023 by the authors. Articles in this book are Open Access and distributed under the Creative Commons Attribution (CC BY) license. The book as a whole is distributed by MDPI under the terms and conditions of the Creative Commons Attribution-NonCommercial-NoDerivs (CC BY-NC-ND) license.

Contents

About the Editor vii

Massimiliano Creta, Giuseppe Celentano, Gianluigi Califano, Roberto La Rocca and Nicola Longo
En-bloc Laser Resection of Bladder Tumors: Where Are We Now?
Reprinted from: *J. Clin. Med.* 2022, *11*, 3463, doi:10.3390/jcm11123463 1

Monika Gudowska-Sawczuk, Jacek Kudelski, Michał Olkowicz, Grzegorz Młynarczyk, Piotr Chłosta and Barbara Mroczko
The Clinical Significance of Serum Free Light Chains in Bladder Cancer
Reprinted from: *J. Clin. Med.* 2023, *12*, 3294, doi:10.3390/jcm12093294 5

Rocco Simone Flammia, Antonio Tufano, Francesco Chierigo, Christoph Würnschimmel, Benedikt Hoeh, Gabriele Sorce, et al.
The Effect of Sex on Disease Stage and Survival after Radical Cystectomy in Non-Urothelial Variant-Histology Bladder Cancer
Reprinted from: *J. Clin. Med.* 2023, *12*, 1776, doi:10.3390/jcm12051776 15

Krystian Kaczmarek, Artur Lemiński, Bartosz Małkiewicz, Adam Gurwin, Janusz Lisiński and Marcin Słojewski
Diminishing the Gender-Related Disparity in Survival among Chemotherapy Pre-Treated Patients after Radical Cystectomy—A Multicenter Observational Study
Reprinted from: *J. Clin. Med.* 2023, *12*, 1260, doi:10.3390/jcm12041260 25

José M. Caballero, José M. Gili, Juan C. Pereira, Alba Gomáriz, Carlos Castillo and Montserrat Martín-Baranera
Risk Factors Involved in the High Incidence of Bladder Cancer in an Industrialized Area in North-Eastern Spain: A Case–Control Study
Reprinted from: *J. Clin. Med.* 2023, *12*, 728, doi:10.3390/jcm12020728 37

Karla Beatríz Peña, Francesc Riu, Josep Gumà, Francisca Martínez-Madueño, Maria José Miranda, Anna Vidal, et al.
Immunohistochemical Algorithm for the Classification of Muscle-Invasive Urinary Bladder Carcinoma with Lymph Node Metastasis: An Institutional Study
Reprinted from: *J. Clin. Med.* 2022, *11*, 7430, doi:10.3390/jcm11247430 49

Daqing Tan, Jinze Li, Tianhai Lin, Ping Tan, Jiapeng Zhang, Qiao Xiong, et al.
Prognostic Utility of the Modified Glasgow Prognostic Score in Urothelial Carcinoma: Outcomes from a Pooled Analysis
Reprinted from: *J. Clin. Med.* 2022, *11*, 6261, doi:10.3390/jcm11216261 61

Antonio Tufano, Nadia Cordua, Valerio Nardone, Raffaele Ranavolo, Rocco Simone Flammia, Federica D'Antonio, et al.
Prognostic Significance of Organ-Specific Metastases in Patients with Metastatic Upper Tract Urothelial Carcinoma
Reprinted from: *J. Clin. Med.* 2022, *11*, 5310, doi:10.3390/jcm11185310 77

Karla B. Peña, Francesc Riu, Anna Hernandez, Carmen Guilarte, Joan Badia and David Parada
Usefulness of the Urine Methylation Test (Bladder EpiCheck®) in Follow-Up Patients with Non-Muscle Invasive Bladder Cancer and Cytological Diagnosis of Atypical Urothelial Cells—An Institutional Study
Reprinted from: *J. Clin. Med.* 2022, *11*, 3855, doi:10.3390/jcm11133855 89

Henglong Hu, Mengqi Zhou, Binrui Yang, Shiwei Zhou, Zheng Liu and Jiaqiao Zhang
A Systematic Review on the Role of Repeat Transurethral Resection after Initial en Bloc Resection for Non-Muscle Invasive Bladder Cancer
Reprinted from: *J. Clin. Med.* **2022**, *11*, 5049, doi:10.3390/jcm11175049 . . . . **99**

Łukasz Nowak, Wojciech Krajewski, Jan Łaszkiewicz, Bartosz Małkiewicz, Joanna Chorbińska, et al.
The Impact of Surgical Waiting Time on Oncological Outcomes in Patients with Upper Tract Urothelial Carcinoma Undergoing Radical Nephroureterectomy: A Systematic Review
Reprinted from: *J. Clin. Med.* **2022**, *11*, 4007, doi:10.3390/jcm11144007 . . . . **117**

About the Editor

Massimiliano Creta

Massimiliano Creta was born in Caserta (Italy) in 1979. In 2004, he graduated with honors in Medicine and Surgery at the University of Campania "Luigi Vanvitelli", and in 2010, he completed, with honors, the residency course in Urology at the University "Federico II" of Naples. In 2013, he received his doctorate in "Surgical Science and Advanced Diagnostic and Therapeutic Technology" at the University "Federico II" of Naples. Since 2018, he has been an Assistant Professor of Urology at the University "Federico II" of Naples (Italian law n. 240/2010—art.24, paragraph 3, lett.a), and he is eligible for Associate Professor of Urology.

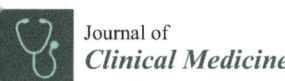

Editorial

En-bloc Laser Resection of Bladder Tumors: Where Are We Now?

Massimiliano Creta *, Giuseppe Celentano, Gianluigi Califano, Roberto La Rocca and Nicola Longo

Department of Neurosciences, Reproductive Sciences and Odontostomatology, University of Naples Federico II, 80130 Naples, Italy; dr.giuseppecelentano@gmail.com (G.C.); gianl.califano2@gmail.com (G.C.); larocca@unina.it (R.L.R.); nicola.longo@unina.it (N.L.)
* Correspondence: massimiliano.creta@unina.it; Tel./Fax: +39-081-7462-611

Transurethral resection of bladder tumors (TURBT) is a crucial procedure in the management of bladder cancer. The goals of TURBT are to make the correct diagnosis, sample the detrusor muscle for staging, and completely remove all visible lesions [1–5]. The quality of the resection strongly influences patient prognosis and overall treatment success. TURBT can be performed by either conventional fractioned or en-bloc techniques. Although it is still the gold standard, conventional TURBT using the incision and scatter technique has a number of potential drawbacks. For example, thermal damage to nearby tissue can lead to difficulty in the pathological evaluation of fragmented tissue, and tumor fragmentation with a high number of exfoliated cancer cells could lead to infield and outfield recurrences [1–5].

First introduced in 1997 by Kawada et al., en-bloc resection of bladder tumors (ERBT) has recently emerged as a promising alternative to conventional TURBT [6]. It involves complete tumor removal and avoids incision through the tumor (a no-touch technique), thus respecting the conventional principles of oncological surgery. Technically, the procedure may be performed with different approaches and energy sources, e.g., knife electrodes, modified J-loops, monopolar or bipolar electrocautery, water jets, or lasers. Laser ERBT involves the use of laser beams to dissect bladder lesions, freeing them from their base and the surrounding tissue. A variety of lasers have been used to perform ERBT, including thulium, holmium, and KTP lasers.

Currently, only few randomized controlled trials have been published comparing laser ERBT to conventional TURBT, with follow-up ranging from 12 to 36 months [1–3]. Overall, laser ERBT appears to be a safer procedure for bladder tumor resection. Indeed, observed intra-and perioperative advantages of laser ERBT include: lower overall complication rates; absent obturator nerve reflexes and a subsequent low incidence of bladder perforation due to the lack of electrical effect; lower rates of post-operative bladder irrigation and lower bladder irrigation times; shorter catheterization times and lengths of hospital stay; and higher rates of the immediate postoperative instillation of chemotherapy [1–3]. A further advantage of laser ERBT includes the potential to perform the procedure without the cessation of anti-platelet or anti-coagulant drugs. One study found higher operative times with laser ERBT mainly due to the higher precision of resection and to the longer time needed for the laser treatment of anterior wall large tumors [2].

Based on the results from the pathological examination of tumor specimens, laser ERBT fulfills the oncological criteria of optimized resection with low residual tumor rates and improved specimen quality. Indeed, it provides higher detrusor muscle sampling rates (a surrogate marker of TURBT quality), and a lower incidence of residual tumors at re-TURBT [3].

Unfortunately, little evidence exists comparing laser and electrical ERBT. In their multicenter European study, Kramer et al. demonstrate comparable outcomes in terms of operation times, irrigation times, and length of catheterization and hospital stay in patients

Citation: Creta, M.; Celentano, G.; Califano, G.; La Rocca, R.; Longo, N. En-bloc Laser Resection of Bladder Tumors: Where Are We Now? *J. Clin. Med.* 2022, 11, 3463. https://doi.org/10.3390/jcm11123463

Received: 3 June 2022
Accepted: 15 June 2022
Published: 16 June 2022

Publisher's Note: MDPI stays neutral with regard to jurisdictional claims in published maps and institutional affiliations.

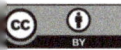

Copyright: © 2022 by the authors. Licensee MDPI, Basel, Switzerland. This article is an open access article distributed under the terms and conditions of the Creative Commons Attribution (CC BY) license (https://creativecommons.org/licenses/by/4.0/).

undergoing electrical and laser ERBT [5]. Detrusor muscle sampling was reported in 96.2% and 100% of specimens following electrical and laser ERBT, respectively [5]. A statistically low incidence of conversion to conventional TURBT, as well a statistically—although not clinically—significant advantage in terms of hemoglobin drop was noted in in patients undergoing laser ERBT [5]. Statistically insignificant differences were noted in terms of operation times, irrigation times, and length of catheterization and hospital stay. Detrusor muscle sampling was reported in 96.2% and 100% of specimens following electrical and laser ERBT, respectively [5]. Statistically insignificant differences in terms of recurrence rates were noted at the 12-month follow-up [5]. From a technical point of view, the authors consider the ability to cut a precise line around the tumor and the better vision obtained during laser ERBT as an advantage primarily for larger tumors [5]. On the other hand, however, switching from ERBT to conventional TURBT is easier when an electrical device is already being used [5].

A more recent study comparing monopolar, bipolar, and thulium laser ERBT confirmed similar rates of detrusor muscle sampling in the specimens and significantly lower rates of the obturator nerve reflex [6]. Out of six conversions to conventional TURBT, bladder cancer was found on the anterior wall and dome in five cases, and in the proximity of the meatus in one case [6]. Therefore, given the high rate of conversion for lesions in the anterior wall, the authors suggest a preference for electrical energy in these cases to avoid the increased potential risk of changing instruments and the subsequent waste of surgical material [6].

Despite promising preliminary evidence regarding laser ERBT, a number of issues remain under debate and under investigation.

Tumor selection criteria are still unconfirmed. Although it is estimated that ERBT is not feasible for almost 30% of tumors due to size, morphology, and/or location, laser ERBT has been performed for tumors up to 4.5–5.5 cm in diameter and in virtually all locations throughout the bladder [3,4].

Additionally, the risks associated with prolonged operative times, mainly in older patients, should be carefully evaluated.

Although the thulium–yttrium–aluminum–garnet laser is considered the device of choice by some authors when performing ERBT, due to its minimal penetration depth and decreased peak power, the search for a more efficient laser to perform ERBT deserves further investigation [7].

Finally, although insignificant differences in terms of recurrence rate have been found by some authors, most studies are not able to find differences in recurrence-free survival as the length of follow-up is still suboptimal, and long-term follow-ups are awaited.

Author Contributions: Conceptualization, M.C. and N.L.; writing—original draft preparation, M.C. and G.C. (Giuseppe Celentano); writing—review and editing, G.C. (Gianluigi Califano) and R.L.R. All authors have read and agreed to the published version of the manuscript.

Funding: This research received no external funding.

Institutional Review Board Statement: Not applicable.

Informed Consent Statement: Not applicable.

Data Availability Statement: Not applicable.

Conflicts of Interest: The authors declare no conflict of interest.

References

1. Liu, H.; Wu, J.; Xue, S.; Zhang, Q.; Ruan, Y.; Sun, X.; Xia, S. Comparison of the safety and efficacy of conventional monopolar and 2-micron laser transurethral resection in the management of multiple nonmuscle-invasive bladder cancer. *J. Int. Med. Res.* **2013**, *41*, 984–992. [CrossRef]
2. Chen, X.; Liao, J.; Chen, L.; Qiu, S.; Mo, C.; Mao, X.; Yang, Y.; Zhou, S.; Chen, J. En bloc transurethral resection with 2-micron continuous-wave laser for primary non-muscle-invasive bladder cancer: A randomized controlled trial. *World J. Urol.* **2015**, *33*, 989–995. [CrossRef] [PubMed]

Hashem, A.; Mosbah, A.; El-Tabey, N.A.; Laymon, M.; Ibrahiem, E.H.; Elhamid, M.A.; Elshal, A.M. Holmium Laser En-bloc Resection Versus Conventional Transurethral Resection of Bladder Tumors for Treatment of Non-muscle-invasive Bladder Cancer: A Randomized Clinical Trial. *Eur. Urol. Focus* **2021**, *7*, 1035–1043. [CrossRef]

Croghan, S.M.; Compton, N.; Manecksha, R.P.; Cullen, I.M.; Daly, P.J. En bloc transurethral resection of bladder tumors: A review of current techniques. *Can. Urol. Assoc. J.* **2022**, *16*, E287–E293. [CrossRef] [PubMed]

Kramer, M.W.; Rassweiler, J.J.; Klein, J.; Martov, A.; Baykov, N.; Lusuardi, L.; Janetschek, G.; Hurle, R.; Wolters, M.; Abbas, M.; et al. En bloc resection of urothelium carcinoma of the bladder (EBRUC): A European multicenter study to compare safety, efficacy, and outcome of laser and electrical en bloc transurethral resection of bladder tumor. *World J. Urol.* **2015**, *33*, 1937–1943. [CrossRef]

Diana, P.; Gallioli, A.; Fontana, M.; Territo, A.; Bravo, A.; Piana, A.; Baboudjian, M.; Gavrilov, P.; Rodriguez-Faba, Ó.; Gaya, J.M.; et al. Energy source comparison in en-bloc resection of bladder tumors: Subanalysis of a single-center prospective randomized study. *World J. Urol.* **2022**, *31*, 1–7. [CrossRef]

Enikeev, D.; Babjuk, M.; Shpikina, A.; Shariat, S.; Glybochko, P. En bloc resection for nonmuscle-invasive bladder cancer: Selecting a proper laser. *Curr. Opin. Urol.* **2022**, *32*, 173–178. [CrossRef] [PubMed]

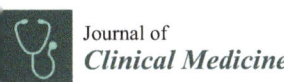

Article

The Clinical Significance of Serum Free Light Chains in Bladder Cancer

Monika Gudowska-Sawczuk [1,*], Jacek Kudelski [2], Michał Olkowicz [2], Grzegorz Młynarczyk [2], Piotr Chłosta [3,4] and Barbara Mroczko [5]

1. Department of Biochemical Diagnostics, Medical University of Bialystok, Waszyngtona 15A St., 15-269 Bialystok, Poland
2. Department of Urology, Medical University of Bialystok, M. Skłodowskiej-Curie 24A St., 15-276 Bialystok, Poland
3. Department of Urology, Jagiellonian University Medical College, Jakubowskiego 2 St., 30-688 Kraków, Poland
4. Department of Urology, Medical University of Vienna, Währinger Gürtel 18-20 St., 1090 Vienna, Austria
5. Department of Neurodegeneration Diagnostics, Medical University of Bialystok, Waszyngtona 15A St., 15-269 Bialystok, Poland
* Correspondence: monika.gudowska-sawczuk@umb.edu.pl; Tel.: +48-85-831-8703

Abstract: This research aimed to assess the clinical usefulness of serum kappa (κ) and lambda (λ) free light chains (FLCs) in patients with bladder cancer (BC). One hundred samples were collected and analysed from healthy volunteers (C) and bladder cancer patients. Cancer patients were divided into two subgroups: low-grade (LG) and high-grade cancer (HG). Concentrations of FLCs, CEA, CA19-9, creatinine and urea were measured per manufacturers' guidelines. The concentrations of κ and λ FLCs and CEA were significantly higher in BC patients in comparison to the control group. Moreover, the concentrations of κ and λ FLCs and CEA were significantly higher in both low-grade as well as high-grade cancer in comparison to the controls. The levels of κ and λ FLCs differed between tumour grades, with patients presenting higher concentrations in high-grade compared to low-grade cancer. In the total study group, κFLC correlated with λFLC, the κ:λ ratio, CRP, CEA, CA19-9, creatinine and urea. There was also a correlation between λFLC and κFLC, CRP, CEA, creatinine and urea. The λFLC showed a higher ability (sensitivity and PPV) to detect bladder cancer in comparison to κFLC and CEA. In addition, λFLC had a higher ability to exclude BC (specificity and NPV) than κFLC and CEA. λFLC also showed the highest accuracy in the detection of bladder cancer. In conclusion, the revealed differences in the concentrations of both κ and λ FLCs suggest their potential participation in bladder cancer development. Increased concentrations of free light chains in bladder cancer patients and the association with the tumour grade suggest that κ and λ FLC measurements may be useful in the diagnosis and prognosis of bladder cancer. This is the first research that evaluates the concentration of FLCs in bladder cancer, so further studies are necessary to confirm their usefulness as tumour markers of this malignancy.

Keywords: free light chains; FLC; kappa; lambda; cancer; bladder cancer; biomarker

1. Introduction

Bladder cancer (BC) is one of the most common urogenital cancers with a high mortality rate. The bladder cancer development risk is almost four times higher among men than women [1]. The list of risk factors includes, for example, smoking, type 2 diabetes, the exposure of the bladder area to ionizing radiation and the chronic inflammation of the bladder. Moreover, the chance of bladder cancer increases with age, and nearly 70% of diagnosed patients are people aged 65 and higher [2–4]. The most common BC symptoms are the appearance of painless, but massive, hematuria; the urgent need to pass urine; and pollakiuria.

Currently, the diagnosis of bladder cancer includes ultrasound examination, cystoscopy and the invasive puncturing of suspicious sites for histopathological examination. Urine cytology is recommended as a supplement to cystoscopy, but the diagnostic specificity of urine cytology is high only in high-grade bladder cancer. On the other hand, a negative result does not exclude the presence of cancer. Unfortunately, the possibilities of laboratory diagnostics concerning bladder cancer are limited. Thus, finding a quick and easy non-invasive biomarker seems to be very important because the timing of the diagnosis is crucial in further treatment, prognosis and patient survival [5–7].

Local inflammation, which may spread throughout the body, is associated with the presence of factors that trigger the immune system's response. In addition to infections or tissue damage, tumours may also cause inflammation [8]. In the course of cancer and other inflammatory conditions, increased immunoglobulin synthesis is observed very often. Additionally, the production of antibodies is always accompanied by a slight excess synthesis of the kappa (κ) and lambda (λ) immunoglobulin light chains, which are not bound to the heavy chain. Small amounts of free light chains (FLCs) are released into peripheral and may also be found in various body fluids such as urine. They are quickly filtered by the glomeruli andare normally present in the urine only in trace amounts. Physiologically, approximately 500 mg per day of FLCs are produced with a $\kappa{:}\lambda$ ratio equal to approximately 2:1. At the time of the excessive production of FLCs, the reabsorption capacity of the renal tubules may be exceeded, resulting in the accumulation of FLCs in the serum [9,10]. This can occur in many clinical conditions, including chronic inflammation, immunological disorders, kidney failure and cancer. Increased levels of FLCs have been observed in different body fluids of patients with, e.g., multiple sclerosis and breast, lung or gastric cancers [11–15]. However, it should be noted that, as far as we are aware, serum FLCs have never been evaluated in the samples of patients with bladder cancer. Therefore, this study aimed to assess the significance and diagnostic utility of free light chains in bladder cancer.

2. Material and Methods

2.1. Study Design

We performed a research study involving patients with bladder cancer and healthy volunteers. Samples were collected between May 2022 and December of the same year. Each participant in the study had their kappa and lambda free light chain concentrations measured. At the same time, we determined the concentrations of CEA and CA19-9 as comparative markers. Then, we compared the results of the tested parameters between healthy controls and patients with bladder cancer and between different stages of cancer.

2.2. Subjects

Patients with bladder cancer were admitted to the Department of Urology of the Medical University of Bialystok. Subsequently, 60 patients who were referred for further transurethral resection of bladder tumour (TURBT) were enrolled in this study. Patients included in the study had a bladder tumour detected by cystoscopy and ultrasound. Fourteen patients had TURBT in the past. No other active cancer diseases were found. Tumour staging and classification were conducted per European Association of Urology guidelines. Patients with bladder cancer were divided into two subgroups: low-grade (n = 52%) and high-grade (n = 48%). In addition, according to the depth of tumour invasion (T) three groups of patients were distinguished: Ta (52%), T1 (15%) and T2 (23%).

Tested patients were males (n = 45) and females (n = 15) (age range: 56–80, mean age: 66.8).

The diagnosis of bladder cancer was based on the patient's symptoms, ultrasound examination, cystoscopy and the result of the histopathological examination.

2.3. Control Group

Overall, 40 healthy volunteers (males $n = 19$, females $n = 21$) were admitted to our institution as the control group (age range: 23–75, mean age: 48.3). For each potential participant in the control group, the following exclusion criteria were applied: other comorbidities that can affect free light chain concentrations; pathological changes in the urinary system; active infections, both viral and bacterial.

Informed consent was obtained from all patients with bladder cancer and healthy volunteers. The study was approved on 25 June 2020 by the Bioethical Committee at the Medical University of Bialystok (APK.002.240.220).

2.4. Blood Sampling

Blood specimens were taken by vein puncture. Serum samples were obtained by centrifugation. Then, serum samples were aliquoted and frozen at −80 °C until they were analysed.

2.5. Methods

The concentrations of serum kappa and lambda-free light chains were measured on the Optilite analyser (The Binding Site, Birmingham, UK) with the use of the turbidimetric method. Determinations were performed under the manufacturer's guidelines.

Detection ranges of serum FLCs listed in instructions:

κFLC—2.90–127.00 mg/L;
λFLC—5.20–139.00 mg/L;
κ:λ ratio—0.26–1.65.

Concentrations of CEA, CA19-9, CRP, creatinine and urea were measured on the Alinity analyser (Abbott) following the manufacturer's recommendations. CEA and CA19-9 were assessed using the chemiluminescent microparticle immunoassay (CMIA) method. CRP was measured using the immunoturbidimetric method, and creatinine and urea were measured with the use of the enzymatic method. Detection ranges for the aforementioned parameters were 1.73–1500.00 ng/mL, 2.06–1200.00 U/mL, 1.00–480.00 mg/dL, 2.5–400.00 mg/dL and 3.00–125.00 mg/dL. In cases of concentrations below the lower limit of detection, the lowest values of the detection were used.

2.6. Statistical Analysis

Statistical data analysis has been performed using the Statistica 13.3 analytics software. The Mann–Whitney U test was used for the evaluation of the differences between the tested groups. The Spearman rank correlation test was used to check the association between tested variables. Cut-off values for κFLC, λFLC and CEA were calculated by Youden's index as a criterion for selecting the optimum cut-off points.

p values < 0.05 were considered statistically significant.

3. Results

3.1. Patients' Ages

The ages of the control group's participants were significantly lower than the ages of the patients with bladder cancer ($p < 0.005$).

3.2. Serum Concentrations of Free Light Chains and Tumour Markers

The results of serum κ and λ FLCs, the κ:λ ratio, CEA and CA19-9 in the patients with bladder cancer and the healthy controls are presented in Table 1. Figure 1 is the visual presentation of the serum concentrations of FLCs as well as the κ:λ ratio.

The serum concentrations of κFLC and λFLC differed significantly between the tested groups ($p < 0.001$ for both). Similarly to the κFLC and λFLC concentrations, the level of CEA was significantly higher in bladder cancer patients in comparison to the healthy controls ($p < 0.001$). The values of the κ:λ ratio and CA19-9 were similar in the bladder cancer patients and the controls ($p = 0.661$ and $p = 0.206$, respectively).

Table 1. The results of serum κ and λ FLCs, the κ:λ ratio, CEA and CA19-9 in patients with bladder cancer and healthy controls.

	Variable Tested	κFLC [mg/L]	λFLC [mg/L]	κ:λ Ratio	CEA [ng/mL]	CA19-9 [U/mL]
Bladder cancer (A)	Median (min–max values).	23.09 [B]* (11.50–137.00)	18.98 [B]* (7.36–55.10)	1.17 (0.82–3.26)	2.60 [B]* (1.72–18.83)	7.34 (2.05–256.43)
Control group (B)		12.36 [A]* (6.28–23.70)	10.86 [A]* (6.84–22.00)	1.22 (0.51–1.77)	1.73 [A]* (0.66–4.60)	4.18 (2.06–19.38)

[A], Bladder cancer; [B], control group; *—the significant differences between tested groups.

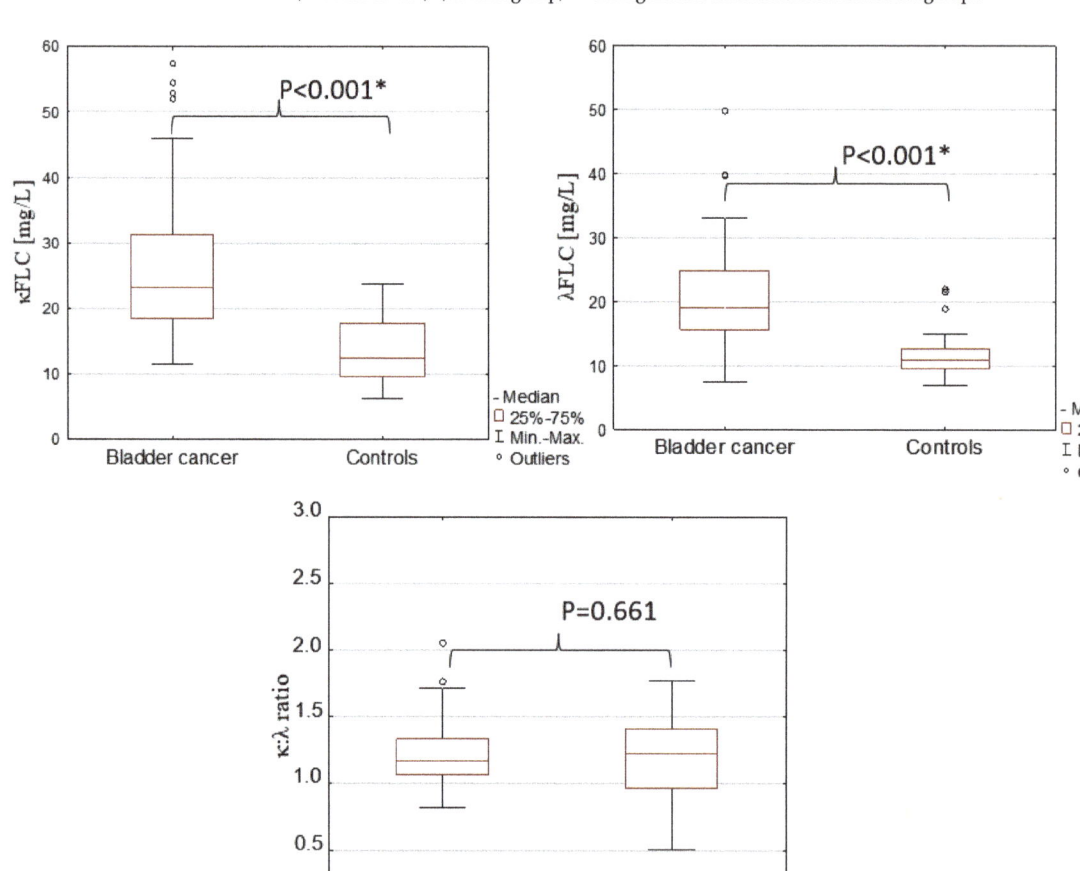

Figure 1. Serum concentrations of FLCs and the κ:λ ratio in patients with bladder cancer and controls *—the significant differences between tested groups.

The statistical analysis revealed that the median serum concentrations of κFLC and λFLC depend on the tumour grade (Figure 2).

The medians of κFLC and λFLC concentrations were higher in high-grade bladder cancer (25.16 and 21.79 mg/L, respectively) than in low-grade (20.55 and 16.73 mg/L, $p = 0.005$ and $p = 0.027$, respectively). The median value of the κ:λ ratio and the concentra tions of CEA and CA19-9 did not differ between the low (1.16, 2.87 ng/mL and 5.69 U/mL, respectively) and high grades of cancer (1.19, 2.27 ng/mL and 6.37 U/mL, respectively).

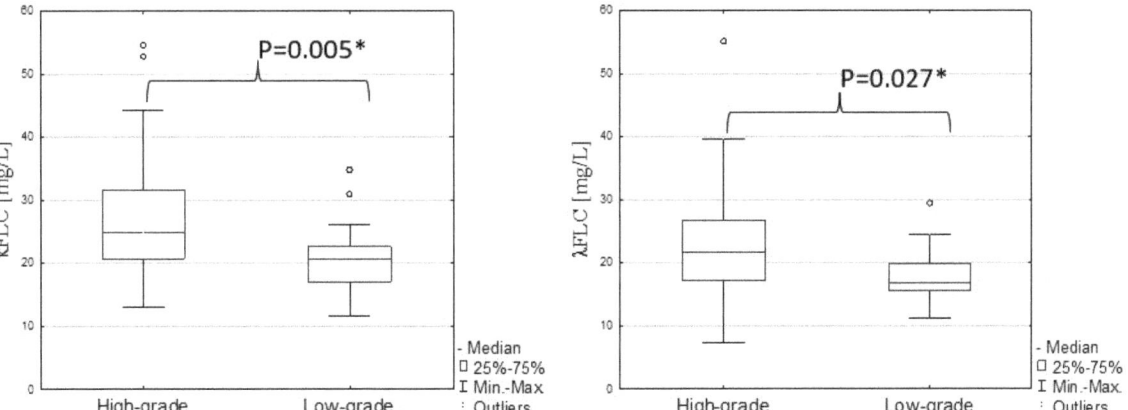

Figure 2. Serum concentrations of κFLC and λFLC in high- and low-grade bladder cancer. *—the significant differences between tested groups.

Moreover, the concentrations of κFLC, λFLC and CEA were significantly lower in the control group in comparison to low- ($p < 0.001$ for all comparisons) and high-grade cancer ($p = 0.017$, $p < 0.001$ and $p < 0.001$, respectively). The concentrations of CA19-9 and the κ:λ ratio did not differ between the control group and low-grade bladder cancer ($p = 0.953$ and $p = 0.732$, respectively) or high-grade bladder cancer ($p = 0.183$ and $p = 0.676$, respectively).

The serum concentrations of the free light chains and CEA according to the tumour infiltration depth (T) are presented in Table 2. The median of κFLC was significantly lower in Ta in comparison to T1 ($p = 0.033$) and T2 ($p = 0.050$). The λFLC concentration differs significantly between Ta and T1 ($p = 0.005$), but there was not any difference between Ta and T2 ($p = 0.357$). The concentrations of κFLC and λFLC were similar between T1 and T2 ($p = 0.703$ and $p = 0.657$, respectively). There was no difference in CEA concentration between Ta and T1 ($p = 0.475$), between Ta and T2 ($p = 0.310$) and between T1 and T2 ($p = 0.182$).

Table 2. Serum concentrations of free light chains and CEA according to the tumour infiltration depth (T).

		κFLC [mg/L]	λFLC [mg/L]	CEA [ng/mL]
Ta (A)		19.42 [B,C*] (11.50–52.06)	16.68 [B*] (10.28–33.09)	2.56 [B*] (1.73–12.16)
T1 (B)	Median (min–max values).	23.16 [A*] (15.05–86.27)	21.21 [A*] (12.99–39.80)	3.39 [A*] (1.73–18.83)
T2 (C)		29.86 [A*] (14.47–137.00)	21.71 (7.36–28.44)	1.96 [A*] (1.73–3.42)

[A], Ta; [B], T1; [C], T2. *—the significant differences between tested groups.

3.3. Correlations of Free Light Chains with Other Tested Parameters

Correlations between κFLC, λFLC, κ:λ ratio, CRP, CEA, CA19-9, creatinine and urea are presented in Table 3. Spearman's rank correlation test demonstrated that κFLC correlated with all tested parameters whereas λFLC did not correlate with κ:λ ratio and CA 19-9. κ:λ ratio correlated only with κFLC concentration.

Table 3. Spearman correlations between tested variables in the total study group.

Total Study Group	κFLC	λFLC	κ:λ Ratio	CRP	CEA	CA19-9	Creatinine	Urea
κFLC								
r		0.843	0.311	0.458	0.289	0.319	0.353	0.450
p		<0.001 *	<0.001 *	<0.001 *	0.004 *	0.002 *	0.001 *	<0.001 *
λFLC								
r	0.843		−0.121	0.397	0.272	0.199	0.385	0.350
p	<0.001 *		0.213	<0.001 *	0.007 *	0.052	<0.001 *	0.001 *
κ:λ ratio								
r	0.311	−0.121		0.120	0.047	0.178	−0.003	0.197
p	<0.001 *	0.213		0.272	0.650	0.084	0.977	0.080
CRP								
r	0.458	0.397	0.120		0.226	0.140	0.139	0.165
p	<0.001 *	<0.001 *	0.272		0.035 *	0.198	0.231	0.157
CEA								
r	0.289	0.272	0.047	0.226		0.262	−0.156	−0.111
p	0.004 *	0.007 *	0.650	0.035 *		0.009 *	0.146	0.320
CA19-9								
r	0.319	0.199	0.178	0.140	0.262		0.168	0.212
p	0.002 *	0.052	0.084	0.198	0.009 *		0.120	0.058
Creatinine								
r	0.353	0.385	−0.003	0.139	−0.156	0.168		0.514
p	0.001 *	<0.001 *	0.977	0.231	0.146	0.120		<0.001 *
Urea								
r	0.450	0.350	0.197	0.165	−0.111	0.212	0.514	
p	<0.001 *	0.001 *	0.080	0.157	0.320	0.058	<0.001 *	

Correlation ratio (r): —0.000–0.100; —0.101–0.300; —0.301–0.500; —0.501–0.700; —0.701–0.900.
*—significant correlation between tested variables.

3.4. Diagnostic Power of κ and λ Free Light Chains

The diagnostic usefulness of κFLC, λFLC and CEA in bladder cancer is presented in Table 4. The λFLC and κFLC showed a higher ability to detect bladder cancer (a sensitivity of ~80.00% for both) in comparison to CEA. The λFLC had slightly higher PPV than κFLC and CEA (90.30 vs. 82.80 and 82.50, respectively). λFLC also showed the highest ability to exclude bladder cancer, with an 83.80% specificity and an 88.60% negative predictive value.

Table 4. The diagnostic significance of serum κ and λ FLCs in bladder cancer.

	Cut-Off from the ROC	Sensitivity [%]	Specificity [%]	PPV [%]	NPV [%]	ACC [%]
κFLC [mg/L]	16.43	88.30	70.30	82.80	78.80	81.40
λFLC [mg/L]	13.38	93.30	83.80	90.30	88.60	89.70
CEA [ng/mL]	1.74	78.30	65.50	82.50	59.40	74.20

PPV, positive predictive value; NPV, negative predictive value; ACC, accuracy.

The ROC curve analysis indicated that the λFLC showed excellent discrimination ability (AUC = 0.906), whereas the test quality of κFLC and CEA in the detection of bladder cancer was good (Figure 3).

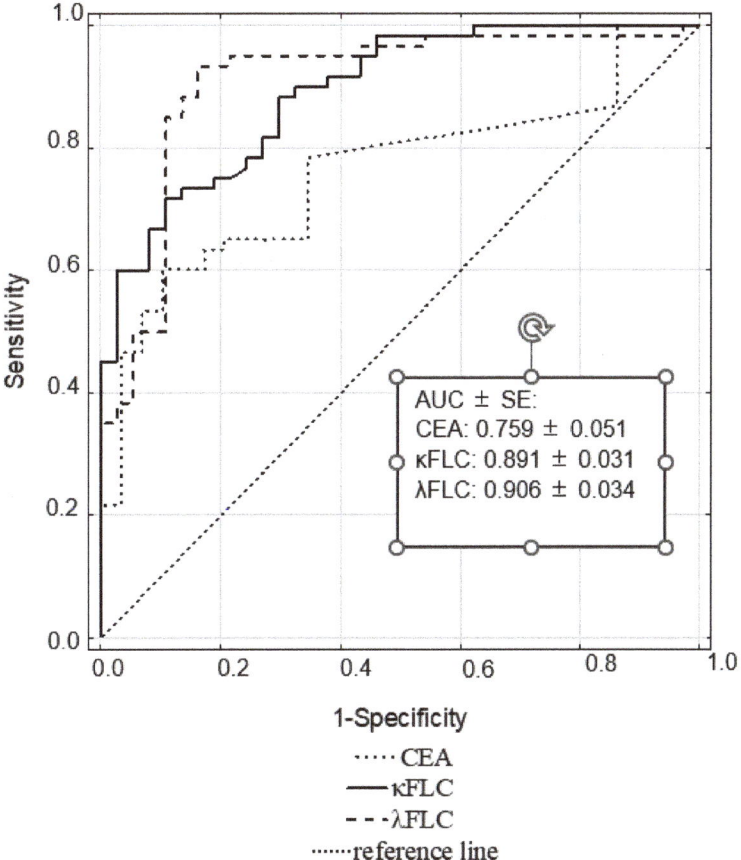

Figure 3. ROC curves for CEA, κ and λ free light chains in bladder cancer.

4. Discussion

When imaging tests (e.g., ultrasound through the abdominal wall) do not show an unequivocal picture of a neoplastic lesion in the bladder, cystoscopy is recommended. It is the most popular diagnostic test for a suspected bladder tumour. The procedure consists of inserting a cystoscope with a vision system through the urethra, which enables the visual assessment of the walls of the bladder and the collection of material for histopathological examination. However, it is an invasive test, and finding non-invasive laboratory markers of bladder cancer is necessary [5,6,16]. The most frequent laboratory test used, both in the diagnosis and in the follow-up of the patient after treatment, is urine sediment cytology. It consists of the microscopic evaluation of the urine sediment obtained from the patient and the detection of exfoliated cancer cells released from the tumour into the lumen of the bladder, which are then excreted in the urine. In recent years, some tumour markers in the urine have also been examined. It has been suggested that, e.g., the nuclear matrix protein 22 (NMP22) BladderChek test may be used for the detection of bladder cancer; however, its sensitivity, specificity and diagnostic usefulness have not been unequivocally confirmed [17,18]. Moreover, the role of blood tumour markers in bladder carcinoma is still not well established. However, carcinoma embryonic antigen (CEA) and carbohydrate antigen 19-9 (CA19-9), for example, have been evaluated in bladder cancer, and it has been observed that their levels correlate with tumour stage and grade.

Despite the significant development of diagnostic methods, there is still a steady increase in the incidence and mortality rates of malignant neoplasms in the world. Therefore, new markers allowing the earlier diagnosis of bladder cancer, more accurate assessments of the disease stage and the better monitoring of therapy is still being sought.

It is known that chronic inflammation underlies many diseases, including malignancies. During immune system activation, in the process of antibody synthesis, free light chains are produced by B lymphocytes. The clinical and diagnostic significance of free light chain measurements in the course of monoclonal gammopathies is currently the best-known and most thoroughly researched method that has been confirmed by numerous studies [19–21]. Additionally, increased levels of FLCs have been observed in the course of, e.g., breast, lung and gastric cancers [12–15]. However, free light chain concentrations, according to our best knowledge, were never evaluated in bladder carcinoma. Thus, all things considered, we decided to evaluate the level of free light chains in the serum of bladder cancer patients.

We have shown that the concentrations of κ and λ FLCs were almost twice as much in the serum of bladder cancer patients as the healthy subjects. On the other hand, the κ:λ ratio did not differ between tested groups, which may suggest the occurrence of polyclonal immunoglobulin FLC synthesis during bladder cancer caused by chronic inflammation. In addition, we observed higher levels of κ and λ FLCs in high-grade bladder cancer so it seems that the concentration of FLCs is associated with tumour grade and disease progression. This may be related to the effect of FLCs on the cells of the immune system. On the other hand, the concentrations of κFLC and λFLC were similar between T1 and T2. However, this may be a result of the unequal distribution of patients in the groups depending on the depth of tumour invasion (T).

It has been observed that many cells of the immune system, including mast cells, enter the tumour microenvironment, and previous studies have shown that mastocytes might be activated by free light chains alone. Mast cells are multifunctional cells that are part of the innate immune system, and they can have anti- and pro-tumorigenic effects. The pro-tumorigenic effects of mast cells include, e.g., their participation in the stimulation of angiogenesis and the degradation of the extracellular matrix, which facilitates the migration of cancer cells and immunosuppression reactions via the secretion of inflammatory factors. Thus, it seems that bladder cancer development may be indirectly related to the level of FLCs, which are over-produced during inflammation and may excessively activate mast cells. Evidence of this may be the presence of free light chains found by other researchers in the areas of mast cell infiltration. On the other hand, the inhibition of FLCs and, as a result, mast cells appears to be a promising therapeutic target for the treatment of cancers [22–26].

Moreover, we observed that FLC concentrations correlate with CRP and CEA levels. Knowing that CRP is a strong reactive acute phase protein and that CEA may be increased in cases of chronic inflammation and cancer, we can conclude that free light chains are closely related to inflammatory responses during bladder cancer progression [27,28]. In addition, the positive correlation between FLCs and elevated levels of creatinine and urea may reflect the obstruction of the flow in the urinary tract caused by cancer.

Among all tested parameters, serum λ and κ free light chain levels had the highest diagnostic value for bladder cancer. Hence, easy-to-perform quantitative measurements of free immunoglobulin light chains may be important blood markers of bladder cancer. We, therefore, carefully suggest that the determination of free light chain concentrations may improve diagnoses and may be used for the differentiation of low- and high-grade bladder cancers.

5. Limitations of the Study

Due to the exclusion criteria applied, the participants in the control group were younger than the patients with bladder cancer. Older patients yield a higher risk of different cancers that may have an impact on, e.g., the CEA concentrations. In addition, some patients also had TURBT in the past, and this should be stated as a limitation and as a possible bias in our study. Moreover, the synthesis of kappa and lambda chains occurs in various inflammatory disorders, so FLC measurements should be taken into consideration not only as a single test but also as a marker of bladder cancer, ultrasound examination and urine cytology. There is a lack of prior research on this topic, so it is hard to understand the role of FLCs in the pathomechanism of bladder cancer development. Because there is no other study that evaluates the usefulness of FLCs in bladder cancer, further studies are needed to confirm their diagnostic and clinical significance.

6. Conclusions

This is the first study that evaluated the significance of serum free light chains in bladder cancer. We showed that the concentrations of free light chains are significantly elevated in bladder cancer and that the levels of κ and λ FLCs increase proportionally with the grade of bladder cancer. In addition, a positive correlation between FLCs with CRP and CEA may reflect the immune system response during cancer development. In conclusion, it seems that serum κ and λ FLCs measurements may be helpful in the diagnosis of bladder cancer with very high diagnostic accuracy.

Author Contributions: Conceptualization, M.G.-S. and B.M.; Methodology, M.G.-S., J.K., M.O., G.M. and P.C.; Formal analysis, M.G.-S.; Investigation, M.G.-S. and M.O.; Data curation, M.G.-S.; Writing—original draft, M.G.-S.; Writing—review & editing, J.K., G.M. and B.M.; Visualization, M.G.-S.; Supervision, B.M.; Funding acquisition, M.G.-S. All authors have read and agreed to the published version of the manuscript.

Funding: This research was funded by Medical University of Bialystok grant number: SUB/1/DN/22/001/2207. The APC was funded by Medical University of Bialystok.

Institutional Review Board Statement: The study was approved on 25 June 2020 by the Bioethical Committee at the Medical Uni-versity of Bialystok (APK.002.240.220).

Informed Consent Statement: Informed consent was obtained from all patients with bladder cancer and healthy volunteers.

Data Availability Statement: The data that support the findings will be available on request under the corresponding author's e-mail: monika.gudowska-sawczuk@umb.edu.pl.

Conflicts of Interest: The authors declare no conflict of interest.

References

1. Dobruch, J.; Daneshmand, S.; Fisch, M.; Lotan, Y.; Noon, A.P.; Resnick, M.J.; Shariat, S.F.; Zlotta, A.R.; Boorjian, S.A. Gender and Bladder Cancer: A Collaborative Review of Etiology, Biology, and Outcomes. *Eur. Urol.* **2016**, *69*, 300–310. [CrossRef]
2. Janković, S.; Radosavljević, V. Risk Factors for Bladder Cancer. *Tumori J.* **2007**, *93*, 4–12. [CrossRef] [PubMed]
3. Letašiová, S.; Medveďová, A.; Šovčíková, A.; Dušinská, M.; Volkovová, K.; Mosoiu, C.; Bartonová, A. Bladder cancer, a review of the environmental risk factors. *Environ. Health* **2012**, *11* (Suppl. S1), S11. [CrossRef]
4. Taylor, J.A.; Kuchel, G.A. Bladder cancer in the elderly: Clinical outcomes, basic mechanisms, and future research direction. *Nat. Rev. Urol.* **2009**, *6*, 135–144. [CrossRef] [PubMed]
5. Shephard, E.; Stapley, S.; Neal, R.D.; Rose, P.; Walter, F.; Hamilton, W.T. Clinical features of bladder cancer in primary care. *Br. J. Gen. Pract.* **2012**, *62*, e598–e604. [CrossRef] [PubMed]
6. Zhu, C.-Z.; Ting, H.-N.; Ng, K.-H.; Ong, T.-A. A review on the accuracy of bladder cancer detection methods. *J. Cancer* **2019**, *10*, 4038–4044. [CrossRef]
7. DeGeorge, K.C.; Holt, H.R.; Hodges, S.C. Bladder Cancer: Diagnosis and Treatment. *Am. Fam. Physician* **2017**, *96*, 507–514.
8. Greten, F.R.; Grivennikov, S.I. Inflammation and Cancer: Triggers, Mechanisms, and Consequences. *Immunity* **2019**, *51*, 27–41. [CrossRef]
9. Jenner, E. Serum free light chains in clinical laboratory diagnostics. *Clin. Chim. Acta* **2014**, *427*, 15–20. [CrossRef]
10. Tosi, P.; Tomassetti, S.; Merli, A.; Polli, V. Serum free light-chain assay for the detection and monitoring of multiple myeloma and related conditions. *Ther. Adv. Hematol.* **2012**, *4*, 37–41. [CrossRef]
11. Gudowska-Sawczuk, M.; Tarasiuk, J.; Kułakowska, A.; Kochanowicz, J.; Mroczko, B. Kappa Free Light Chains and IgG Combined in a Novel Algorithm for the Detection of Multiple Sclerosis. *Brain Sci.* **2020**, *10*, 324. [CrossRef] [PubMed]
12. Gudowska-Sawczuk, M.; Mroczko, B. Free Light Chains as a Novel Diagnostic Biomarker of Immune System Abnormalities in Multiple Sclerosis and HIV Infection. *BioMed Res. Int.* **2019**, *2019*, 8382132. [CrossRef] [PubMed]
13. Groot Kormelink, T.; Powe, D.G.; Kuijpers, S.A.; Abudukelimu, A.; Fens, M.H.; Pieters, E.H.; Kassing van der Ven, W.W.; Habashy, H.O.; Ellis, I.O.; Blokhuis, B.R.; et al. Immunoglobulin free light chains are biomarkers of poor prognosis in basal-like breast cancer and are potential targets in tumor-associated inflammation. *Oncotarget* **2014**, *5*, 3159–3167. [CrossRef] [PubMed]

14. Mastroianni, A.; Panella, R.; Morelli, D. Differential diagnosis between bone relapse of breast cancer and lambda light chain multiple myeloma: Role of the clinical biochemist. *Tumori J.* **2019**, *105*, NP17–NP19. [CrossRef]
15. Ma, J.; Jiang, D.; Gong, X.; Shao, W.; Zhu, Z.; Xu, W.; Qiu, X. Free immunoglobulin light chain (FLC) promotes murine colitis and colitis-associated colon carcinogenesis by activating the inflammasome. *Sci. Rep.* **2017**, *7*, 5165. [CrossRef]
16. Sahraeizadeh, A.; Gharibvand, M.M.; Kazemi, M.; Motamedfar, A.; Sametzadeh, M. The role of ultrasound in diagnosis and evaluation of bladder tumors. *J. Fam. Med. Prim. Care* **2017**, *6*, 840–843. [CrossRef]
17. Cho, E.; Bang, C.K.; Kim, H.; Lee, H.K. An ensemble approach of urine sediment image analysis and NMP22 test for detection of bladder cancer cells. *J. Clin. Lab. Anal.* **2020**, *34*, e23345. [CrossRef]
18. Wang, J.; Zhao, X.; Jiang, X.L.; Lu, D.; Yuan, Q.; Li, J. Diagnostic performance of nuclear matrix protein 22 and urine cytology for bladder cancer: A meta-analysis. *Diagn. Cytopathol.* **2022**, *50*, 300–312. [CrossRef]
19. Milani, P.; Palladini, G.; Merlini, G. Serum-free light-chain analysis in diagnosis and management of multiple myeloma and related conditions. *Scand. J. Clin. Lab. Investig.* **2016**, *76*, S113–S118. [CrossRef]
20. Gran, C.; Afram, G.; Liwing, J.; Verhoek, A.; Nahi, H. Involved free light chain: An early independent predictor of response and progression in multiple myeloma. *Leuk. Lymphoma* **2021**, *62*, 2227–2234. [CrossRef]
21. Silva, C.; Costa, A.; Paiva, D.; Freitas, S.; Alves, G.; Cotter, J. Light-Chain Multiple Myeloma: A Diagnostic Challenge. *Cureus* **2021**, *13*, e19131. [CrossRef] [PubMed]
22. Choi, H.W.; Naskar, M.; Seo, H.K.; Lee, H.W. Tumor-Associated Mast Cells in Urothelial Bladder Cancer: Optimizing Immuno-Oncology. *Biomedicines* **2021**, *9*, 1500. [CrossRef] [PubMed]
23. Lichterman, J.N.; Reddy, S.M. Mast Cells: A New Frontier for Cancer Immunotherapy. *Cells* **2021**, *10*, 1270. [CrossRef] [PubMed]
24. Maciel, T.; Moura, I.; Hermine, O. The role of mast cells in cancers. *F1000Prime Rep.* **2015**, *7*, 9. [CrossRef]
25. Redegeld, F.A.; Thio, M.; Kormelink, T.G. Polyclonal Immunoglobulin Free Light Chain and Chronic Inflammation. *Mayo Clin. Proc.* **2012**, *87*, 1032–1033. [CrossRef]
26. Mortaz, E.; Adcock, I.M.; Jammati, H.; Khosravi, A.; Movassaghi, M.; Garssen, J.; Mogadam, M.A.; Redegeld, F.A. Immunoglobulin Free Light Chains in the Pathogenesis of Lung Disorders. *Iran. J. Allergy Asthma Immunol.* **2017**, *16*, 282–288.
27. Jain, S.; Gautam, V.; Naseem, S. Acute-phase proteins: As diagnostic tool. *J. Pharm. Bioallied Sci.* **2011**, *3*, 118–127. [CrossRef]
28. Hall, C.; Clarke, L.; Pal, A.; Buchwald, P.; Eglinton, T.; Wakeman, C.; Frizelle, F. A Review of the Role of Carcinoembryonic Antigen in Clinical Practice. *Ann. Coloproctol.* **2019**, *35*, 294–305. [CrossRef]

Disclaimer/Publisher's Note: The statements, opinions and data contained in all publications are solely those of the individual author(s) and contributor(s) and not of MDPI and/or the editor(s). MDPI and/or the editor(s) disclaim responsibility for any injury to people or property resulting from any ideas, methods, instructions or products referred to in the content.

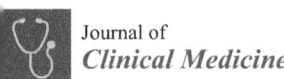

Journal of
Clinical Medicine

Article

The Effect of Sex on Disease Stage and Survival after Radical Cystectomy in Non-Urothelial Variant-Histology Bladder Cancer

Rocco Simone Flammia [1,2,*], Antonio Tufano [1,3], Francesco Chierigo [2,4], Christoph Würnschimmel [2,5], Benedikt Hoeh [2,6], Gabriele Sorce [2,7], Zhen Tian [2], Umberto Anceschi [8], Costantino Leonardo [1], Francesco Del Giudice [1], Carlo Terrone [4], Antonio Giordano [3,9], Andrea Morrione [3], Fred Saad [2], Shahrokh F. Shariat [10,11,12,13,14,15], Alberto Briganti [7], Francesco Montorsi [7], Felix K. H. Chun [6], Michele Gallucci [1] and Pierre I. Karakiewicz [2]

1. Department of Maternal-Child and Urological Sciences, Policlinico Umberto I Hospital, Sapienza University of Rome, 00161 Rome, Italy
2. Cancer Prognostics and Health Outcomes Unit, Division of Urology, University of Montréal Health Center, Montréal, QC H4A 3J1, Canada
3. Sbarro Institute for Cancer Research and Molecular Medicine, Center for Biotechnology, Department of Biology, College of Science and Technology, Temple University, Philadelphia, PA 19122, USA
4. Department of Surgical and Diagnostic Integrated Sciences (DISC), University of Genova, 16146 Genova, Italy
5. Martini-Klinik Prostate Cancer Center, University Hospital Hamburg-Eppendorf, 20251 Hamburg, Germany
6. Department of Urology, University Hospital Frankfurt, Goethe University Frankfurt am Main, 60596 Frankfurt am Main, Germany
7. Division of Experimental Oncology/Unit of Urology, URI, Urological Research Institute, IRCCS San Raffaele Scientific Institute, 20132 Milan, Italy
8. Department of Urology, Regina Elena National Cancer Institute, 00144 Rome, Italy
9. Department of Medical Biotechnology, University of Siena, 53100 Siena, Italy
10. Department of Urology, Weill Cornell Medical College, New York, NY 10065, USA
11. Department of Urology, University of Texas Southwestern, Dallas, TX 75390, USA
12. Department of Urology, Second Faculty of Medicine, Charles University, 128 08 Prague, Czech Republic
13. Institute for Urology and Reproductive Health, I.M. Sechenov First Moscow State Medical University, 119991 Moscow, Russia
14. Hourani Center for Applied Scientific Research, Al-Ahliyya Amman University, Amman 11942, Jordan
15. Department of Urology, Comprehensive Cancer Center, Medical University of Vienna, 1090 Vienna, Austria
* Correspondence: roccosimone92@gmail.com

Abstract: Background: Female sex in patients treated by radical cystectomy (RC) is associated with more advanced stage and worse survival. However, studies supporting these findings mostly or exclusively relied on urothelial carcinoma of the urinary bladder (UCUB) and did not address non-urothelial variant-histology bladder cancer (VH BCa). We hypothesized that female sex is associated with a more advanced stage and worse survival in VH BCa, similarly to that of UCUB. Materials and Methods: Within the SEER database (2004–2016), we identified patients aged ≥18 years, with histologically confirmed VH BCa, and treated with comprehensive RC. Logistic regression addressing the non-organ-confined (NOC) stage, as well as cumulative incidence plots and competing risks regression addressing CSM for females vs. males, were fitted. All analyses were repeated in stage-specific and VH-specific subgroups. Results: Overall, 1623 VH BCa patients treated with RC were identified. Of those, 38% were female. Adenocarcinoma (n = 331, 33%), neuroendocrine tumor (n = 304, 18%), and other VH (n = 317, 37%) were less frequent in females but not squamous cell carcinoma (n = 671, 51%). Across all VH subgroups, female patients had higher NOC rates than males did (68 vs. 58%, p < 0.001), and female sex was an independent predictor of NOC VH BCa (OR = 1.55, p = 0.0001). Overall, five-year cancer-specific mortality (CSM) were 43% for females vs. 34% for males (HR = 1.25, p = 0.02). Conclusion: In VH BC patients treated with comprehensive RC, female sex is associated with a more advanced stage. Independently of stage, female sex also predisposes to higher CSM.

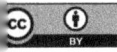

Keywords: muscle-invasive bladder cancer; adenocarcinoma; neuroendocrine carcinoma; variant histology; squamous cell carcinoma; radical cystectomy

1. Introduction

Sex has shown to be an important predictor of survival in urothelial carcinoma of the urinary bladder (UCUB) [1–3]. Specifically, radical cystectomy (RC) in female patients is associated with a more advanced stage and worse survival as compared with males [4–8] However, studies supporting these findings mostly or exclusively relied on UCUB and did not address non-urothelial variant-histology bladder cancer (VH BCa), as reported in a recent systematic review and metanalysis by Uhlig et al. (59 studies, n = 69,666) [9] Consequently, the association between sex and either advanced stage or worse survival in VH Bca treated with RC is unknown. To address this void, we relied on SEER database and examined four VH Bca subgroups: patients with squamous cell carcinoma (SCC), adenocarcinoma (ADK), neuroendocrine carcinoma (NE) and other types (other VH), according to the 2016 World Health Organization (WHO) classification [10,11]. Mixed histology is not coded in the SEER database; thus, these criteria reflect the predominant histologic subtype [12]. We hypothesized that female sex is associated with a more advanced stage and worse survival in VH BCa, similar to that of UCUB.

2. Materials and Methods

2.1. Study Population

Within the SEER database (2004–2016), we identified radical cystectomy (RC) patients aged $\geq$ 18 years old, with a histologically confirmed diagnosis of BCa (International Classification of Disease for Oncology site code C67.0-9), and no distant metastasis according to the American Joint Committee on Cancer (AJCC), Seventh Edition. Only patients harboring VH BCa, consisting of either SCC, ADK, NE, and other types (other VH), were included Moreover, in accord with previous methodology [8], only patients with comprehensive RC that included lymphadenectomy were selected [13]. Patients with disease confirmed by autopsy, death certificate-only cases, and patients exposed to radiotherapy were excluded

2.2. Statistical Analysis

The analysis consisted of two main parts. First, we examined the association between female sex and non-organ-confined stage (NOC = T3-4 and/or N1-3) in univariable and multivariable logistic regression models (LRM) after adjustments for age. All analyses were then repeated in each of four VH-specific subgroups: SCC, ADK, NE, and other VH.

Second, we focused on cancer-specific mortality (CSM) according to female sex and relied on cumulative incidence plots and competing risks regression (CRR) models. Covariates consisted of age, T-stage, N-stage, chemotherapy (CHT), and further adjustment for other-cause mortality (OCM) was performed. All analyses were repeated after stratification according to stage-specific (NOC vs. organ-confined [OC]), as well as VH-specific subgroups (SCC, ADK, NE, other VH). All tests were two-sided with a level of significance set at $p < 0.05$ and R software for statistical computing and graphics (version 3.4.3) was used for all analyses.

3. Results

3.1. Descriptive Characteristics of Study Population

Overall, 1623 patients with VH BCa treated with RC were identified (Table 1). Of those, 38% were female. ADK was less frequent in females than in males (n = 331, 33%), NE (n = 304, 18%), and other VH (n = 317, 37%), but SCC was not (n = 671, 51%). No difference in median age was recorded between females vs. males (67 vs. 68 years).

Table 1. Descriptive characteristics of 1623 VH BCa treated with RC patients, according to sex (female vs. male).

Characteristic	n	Overall n = 1623	Females n = 621 (38%)	Males n = 1002 (62%)	p-Value [2]
Age	1623	67 (58–75) [1]	67 (57–75) [1]	68 (59–75) [1]	0.084
Histological Variants [3]	1623				<0.001
Squamous		671 (41%)	340 (51%)	331 (49%)	
Adenocarcinoma		331 (20%)	109 (33%)	222 (67%)	
Neuroendocrine		304 (19%)	55 (18%)	249 (82%)	
Other		317 (20%)	117 (37%)	200 (63%)	
T-stage	1623				0.001
Ta/Tis		51 (3.1%)	17 (2.7%)	34 (3.4%)	
T1		133 (8.2%)	44 (7.1%)	89 (8.9%)	
T2		492 (30.3%)	159 (25.6%)	333 (33.2%)	
T3-T4		947 (59%)	401 (64%)	546 (54%)	
N-stage	1623				0.3
N+		407 (25%)	165 (27%)	242 (24%)	
Stage	1623				<0.001
Non-organ-confined		100 (62%)	421 (68%)	579 (58%)	
Perioperative Chemotherapy	1623				<0.001
Yes		554 (34.1%)	176 (28.3%)	378 (37.7%)	

[1] Median (IQR), [2] Wilcoxon rank sum test; Pearson's Chi-squared test, [3] Row proportions are reported for each VH according to sex (female vs. male).

3.2. The Association of Sex with Non-Organ-Confined (NOC) VH BCa

Across all VH subtypes (Figure 1), female patients had higher NOC rates than males (68 vs. 58%, $p < 0.001$), and female sex was an independent predictor of NOC VH BCa (OR = 1.55, 95% CI 1.26–1.92, $p < 0.001$).

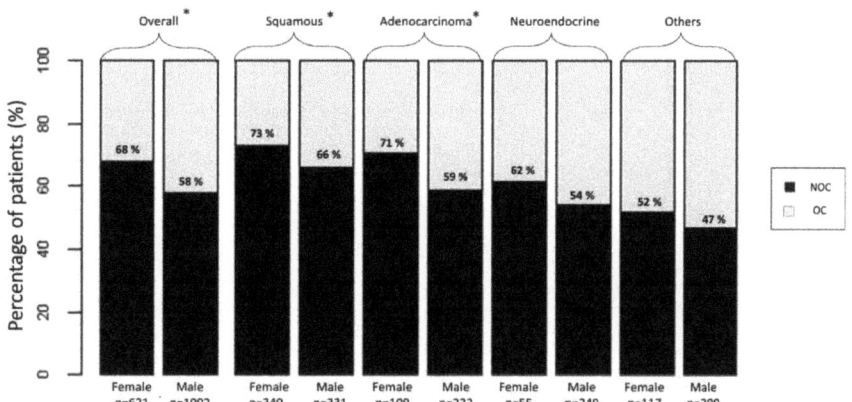

Figure 1. Stacked bar plots depicting stage at presentation according to patient sex in the overall cohort of non-urothelial variant-histology bladder cancer (VH BCa) treated with radical cystectomy and within each VH-specific subgroup. Stages were defined as non-organ-confined (NOC) vs. organ-confined (OC). * $p < 0.05$.

After stratification according to VH-specific subgroups (Figure 1), female patients exhibited higher NOC rates in SCC (73% vs. 66%, $p = 0.046$) and ADK (71% vs. 59%, $p = 0.040$). In SCC and ADK subgroups, female sex was also an independent predictor of NOC VH BCa (Table 2). Conversely, no differences in NOC rates between females and males were detected in NE (62% vs. 54%, $p = 0.3$) and other VH (52% vs. 47%, $p = 0.4$). In NE and other VH, female sex was also not an independent predictor of NOC VH BCa (Table 2).

Table 2. Multivariable logistic regression models predicting non-organ-confined (NOC) stage and multivariable competing risks regression models predicting cancer-specific mortality (CSM) according to sex (female vs. male) in the overall cohort of non-urothelial variant-histology bladder cancer (VH BCa) and within VH-specific subgroup: squamous cell carcinoma (SCC), adenocarcinoma (ADK), neuroendocrine tumor (NE), and other VHs.

	Multivariable Logistic Regression (Non-Organ-Confined, NOC)		Multivariable Competing Risks Regression (Cancer-Specific Mortality, CSM)		
		OR (95%CI)	p-Value		HR (95%CI)	p-Value
Overall cohort	(n = 1623) Females	1.55 (1.26–1.92)	0.0001	(n = 1623) Females	1.25 (1.04–1.50)	0.02
Stage-specific subgroup analyses				OC (n = 623) Females	1.65 (1.08–2.52)	0.02
				NOC (n = 1000) Females	1.17 (0.96–1.43)	0.1
VH-specific subgroup analyses	SCC (n = 671) Females	1.40 (1.01–1.95)	0.047	SCC (n = 671) Females	1.33 (1.01–1.75)	0.045
	ADK (n = 331) Females	1.66 (1.02–2.74)	0.044	ADK (n = 331) Females	1.39 (0.94–2.06)	0.1
	NE (n = 304) Females	1.38 (0.76–2.55)	0.3	NE (n = 304) Females	1.24 (0.77–2.00)	0.4
	Other VH (n = 317) Females	1.29 (0.81–2.06)	0.3	Other VH (n = 317) Females	1.06 (0.69–1.63)	0.8

3.3. Effect of Female Sex in Cancer-Specific Mortality (CSM)

3.3.1. CSM in the Overall Cohort

Across all VH subtypes (n = 1623), five-year CSM rates were 43% for females vs. 34% for males (Figure 2). This translated into a CRR HR of 1.25 (95% CI 1.04–1.50, p = 0.02) after adjustment for age, T-stage, N-stage, VH, CHT, and OCM (Table 2).

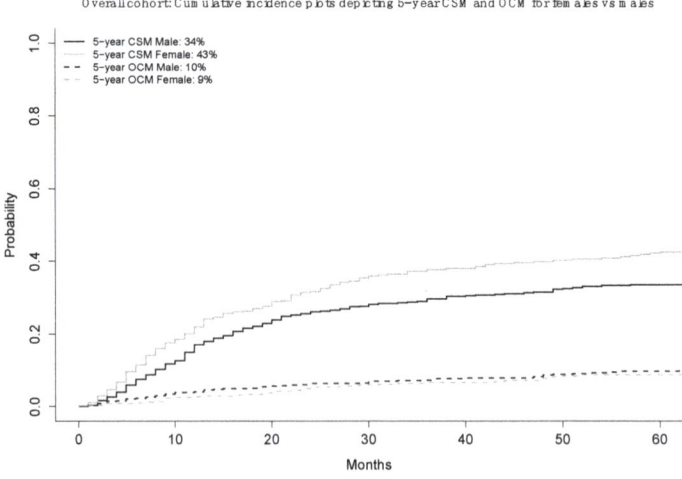

Figure 2. Cumulative incidence plots depicting 5-year cancer-specific mortality (CSM) and 5-year other-cause mortality (OCM) in the overall cohort of non-urothelial variant-histology bladder cancer (VH BCa) according to sex (female vs. male).

3.3.2. CSM according to Stage-Specific Subgroups (OC vs. NOC)

In the OC subgroup (n = 623), five-year CSM rates were 21% for females vs. 15 % for males (Figure 3a). This translated into a CRR HR of 1.65 (95% CI 1.08–2.52, p = 0.02) after adjustment for age, T-stage, VH, CHT, and OCM (Table 2). In the NOC subgroup (n = 1000), five-year CSM rates were 54% for females vs. 48% for males (Figure 3b). This translated into a CRR HR of 1.17 (95% CI 0.96–1.43, p = 0.1) after adjustment for age, T-stage, N-stage, VH, CHT, and OCM (Table 2).

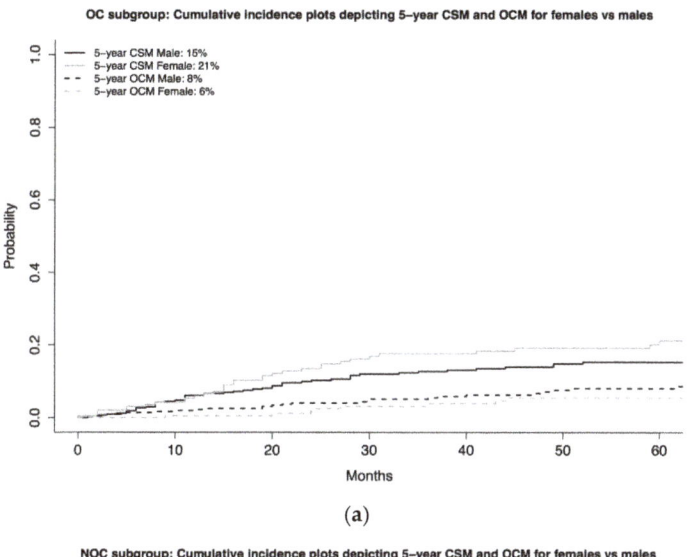

(a)

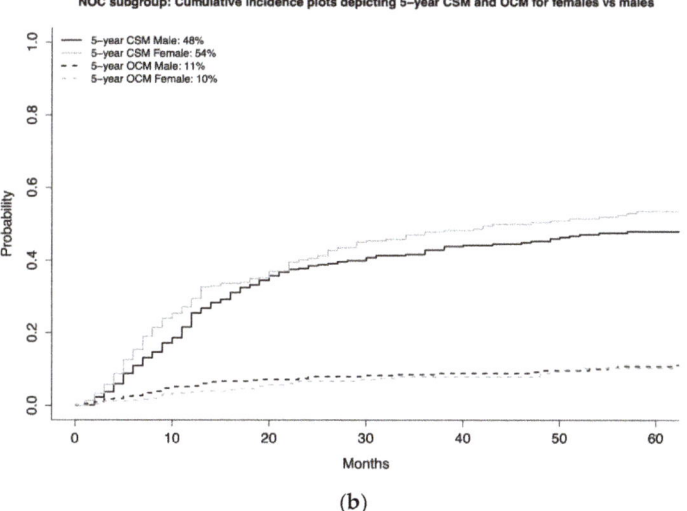

(b)

Figure 3. Cumulative incidence plots depicting 5-year cancer-specific mortality (CSM) and 5-year other-cause mortality (OCM) according to sex (female vs. male) in both the organ-confined (OC) (**a**) as well as non-organ-confined (NOC) subgroup (**b**).

3.3.3. CSM according to VH-Specific Subgroups (SCC, ADK, NE, other VH)

In the SCC subgroup (n = 671), five-year CSM rates were 39% for females vs. 33% for males (Figure 4). This translated into a CRR HR of 1.33 (95% CI 1.01–1.75, p = 0.045), after adjustment for age, T-stage, N-stage, age, and OCM (Table 2).

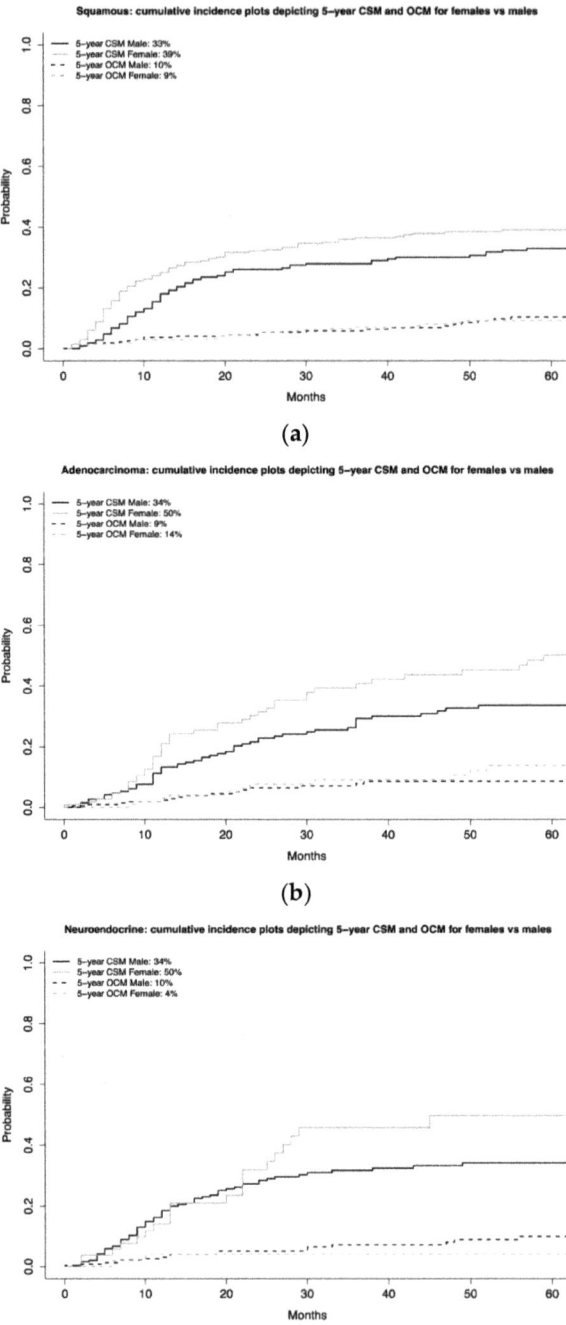

Figure 4. Cont.

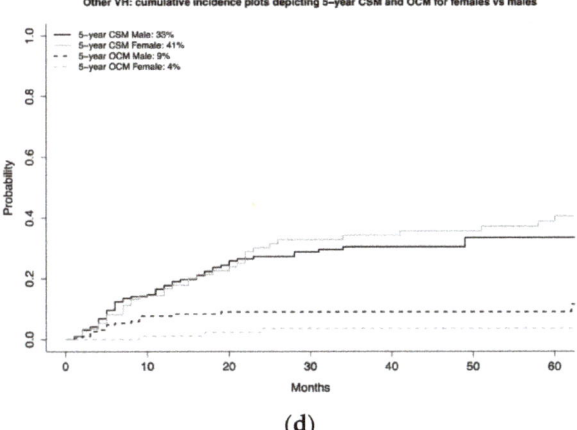

Figure 4. Cumulative incidence plots depicting 5-year cancer-specific mortality (CSM) and 5-year other-cause mortality (OCM), according to sex (female vs. male) in squamous cell carcinoma (SCC) (**a**), adenocarcinoma (ADK) (**b**), neuroendocrine tumor (NE) (**c**), and other VH subgroups (**d**).

In the ADK subgroup ($n = 331$), five-year CSM rates were 50% for females vs. 34% for males (Figure 4). This translated into a CRR HR of 1.39 (95% CI 0.94–2.06, $p = 0.1$) after adjustment for age, T-stage, N-stage, and OCM (Table 2). In the NE subgroup ($n = 304$), five-year CSM rates were 50% for females vs. 34% for males (Figure 4). This translated into a CRR HR of 1.24 (95% CI 0.77–2.00, $p = 0.4$) after adjustment for age, T-stage, N-stage, CHT, and OCM (Table 2). In the other VH subgroup ($n = 317$), five-year CSM rates were 41% for females vs. 33% for 142 males (Figure 4). This translated into a CRR HR of 1.06 (95% CI 0.69–1.63, $p = 0.8$) after adjustment for age, T-stage, N-stage, and OCM (Table 2).

4. Discussion

We hypothesized that female sex is associated with both pathologic stage and CSM in patients with VH BCa treated with comprehensive RC. Moreover, we tested whether CSM sex-related differences also apply to stage-specific and/or VH-specific subgroups. We tested these three hypotheses and observed important sex-related differences.

First, we identified 1623 patients with VH BCa treated with RC. Of those, 38% were females. Females were a minority in ADK (33%) and NE (18%), as well as other VHs (37%) but not in SCC (51%). These observations, except for SCC, agree with findings on UCUB treated with comprehensive RC, where Rosiello et al. reported a 23% female sex prevalence (SEER 2004–2016) [8]. Interestingly, recurrent urinary tract infections (UTIs) are a risk factor for SCC [14], and females are at increased risk of recurrent UTIs in comparison with males. Consequently, the prevalence of recurrent UTIs among females may represent an explanation for the high rate of SCC. We also observed sex-specific stage distribution differences. Specifically, females had NOC VH BCa more frequently than males when all VH patients were assessed (68% vs. 58%), as well as in SCC (73 vs. 66%) and ADK (71 vs. 59%) subgroups, but not in NE (62 vs. 54%) and other VH (52% vs. 47%) subgroups. Moreover, female sex was an independent predictor of NOC in the overall VH BCa cohort (OR 1.55, $p = 0.0001$), as well as in SCC (OR 1.40, $p = 0.047$) and ADK (OR 1.66, $p = 0.044$) subgroups, but not in NE (OR 1.38, $p = 0.3$) and other VH (OR 1.29, $p = 0.3$). Taken together, females represent a minority in VH BCa, except for the SCC subgroup where their proportion is virtually equally to that of males. However, females had NOC VH BCa more frequently than their male counterparts.

Second, we examined the association between female sex and CSM. Here, we accounted for other-cause mortality using CRR models to provide the most unbiased estimate of CSM [15]. In the overall VH BCa cohort, female sex was associated with higher CSM

(HR 1.25, p = 0.02). In stage-specific subgroup analyses (NOC vs. OC), female sex was an independent predictor of higher CSM in OC (HR 1.65, p = 0.02), but not in NOC (HR 1.17, p = 0.1) subgroups. Finally, in VH-specific subgroup analyses, females exhibited higher five-year CSM rates in SCC (39 vs. 33%), ADK (50 vs. 34%), and NE (50 vs. 34%) subgroups, but not in the other VH (41% vs. 33%) subgroup. These differences translated into a statistically significant CRR HR for females vs. males only in SCC (1.33, p = 0.045). Moreover, a clinically meaningful CRR HR was also recorded in ADK (1.39, p = 0.1) and NE subgroups (1.24, p = 0.4), although both lacked statistical significance. Finally, neither statistically significant nor clinically meaningful differences in CSM were observed in the other VH subgroup (1.06, p = 0.8). These observations indicate that the female sex disadvantage is mostly operational in the OC and SCC subgroups. Moreover, female sex is also disadvantageous with respect to CSM in ADK and NE. However, the small sample size in these two subgroups potentially undermined the statistical significance of these results. The rarity of VH BCa and the even greater rarity of VH BCa-specific subgroups represents a major limiting factor in this part of the analysis.

Stage disadvantage in females may reflect a female-specific delay in BCa diagnosis. Indeed, sex-related differences in referral patterns were reported by Mansson et al. [16]. Specifically, a higher proportion of females vs. males with BCa were referred to a department other than urology (26.9% vs. 3.7%) for an initial hematuria work-up. Similarly, Ark et al. observed that females were less likely than males to be referred to a urologist (OR 0.59) [17]. Moreover, Cohn et al. reported significantly longer delays from initial hematuria diagnosis to urological assessment in females vs. males (85.4 vs. 73.6 days, p < 0.001) [18]. These findings are not surprising, since in females, most general practitioners associate microscopic or even gross hematuria with urinary tract infections [19]. Since delay in diagnosis tends to be greater in females than males, it may be postulated that such delay introduces a stage disadvantage in females, as was observed in the current study. These observations are consistent with previous findings regarding UCUB. Consequently, efforts should be made to maximally reduce or even eliminate diagnostic delays in all females patients at risk of BCa, including VH BCa [20,21]. The female sex disadvantage extends beyond stage at diagnosis. Specifically, female sex is associated with higher CSM after comprehensive RC. The current results validated this hypothesis in the overall VH BCa cohort, including highly statistically significant multivariable CRR HR, even after adjustment for OCM. Similarly, in the stage-specific subgroup analyses, a female-specific CSM disadvantage was observed in OC but not in NOC VH BCa after multivariable adjustments, even for OCM. Finally, in VH-specific subgroup analyses, female sex was associated with a higher CSM in SCC, as evidenced by statistically significant multivariable CRR HR, even after adjustment for OCM. Moreover, in the ADK and NE subgroups, female sex was associated with clinically meaningful higher CSM. However, the small sample size of these VH-specific subgroups undermines the statistical significance of these comparisons. Taken together, female sex clearly predisposes to worse CSM in the overall BCa cohort VH, and this effect is clearly detectable in SCC, ADK, and NE, but not in other VH subgroups.

It is important to emphasize the combined detrimental effect of female sex in both stage distribution (NOC) and CSM in VH BCa. Specifically, in the entire VH BCa cohort, as well as in the SCC subgroup, a highly statistically significant association between female sex and both NOC stage and CSM was observed. In consequence, it may be postulated that in VH BCa, female patients not only present with higher stage but independently of stage, female sex is also disadvantageous with respect to survival. This observation is consistent with the same two-step female disadvantage in UCUB reported by Rosiello et al. [8], where female sex is associated with a more advanced stage at presentation, and fully independently of stage, female sex is also associated with a higher CSM.

To the best of our knowledge, we are the first to report this association in patients with VH BC treated with comprehensive RC. Despite the novelty of our findings, our observations are limited in several regards. First, our findings are based on limited sample size, especially within VH-specific subgroup. However, the current cohort represents the largest group of patients with VH BCa treated with RC. Second, the SEER database does not include detailed preoperative information regarding (1) the time interval from diagnosis to RC, (2) the number of recurrences, (3) the use of intravesical therapy, (4) the number and extent of previous trans-urethral bladder tumor resection (TURBT), (5) TURBT completeness, (6) tumor multifocality, (7) tumor size, (8) presence of associated CIS, and (9) molecular or mutational characteristics, as well as other similar pathological variables that may have been systematically worse in women [22–26]. Third, a centralized pathology review is not available within the SEER database. Fourth, SEER database findings are applicable only to patients from the United States and are not generalizable to other healthcare settings. These, as well as all other limitations related to the retrospective, population-based nature of the SEER database, apply to this research and to other similar analyses that were based on other similar large-scale data repositories (National Cancer Data Base, National Inpatient Sample, SEER-Medicare, or National Surgical Quality Improvement Program).

However, no prospective studies investigating the role of sex in VH BCa treated with RC have been published so far. Consequently, the current findings represent the strongest, more robust, and most generalizable proof of the association of female sex with the outcome of VH BCa treated with RC.

5. Conclusions

In VH BC patients treated with comprehensive RC, female sex is associated with a more advanced stage. Fully independently of stage, female sex is also associated with a higher CSM.

Author Contributions: Conceptualization, P.I.K. and R.S.F. methodology, P.I.K. and R.S.F. software, Z.T., F.C., A.T., G.S., C.W. and B.H.; validation, P.I.K. and C.L.; formal analysis, Z.T.; investigation, U.A. and A.T.; resources, A.G.; data curation, R.S.F.; writing—original draft preparation, R.S.F. and A.T.; writing—review and editing, P.I.K.; visualization, P.I.K., A.M. and A.G.; supervision, S.F.S., P.I.K., A.B., F.M., F.S., F.K.H.C., C.T. and M.G.; project administration, F.D.G.; funding acquisition, F.D.G. and C.L. All authors have read and agreed to the published version of the manuscript.

Funding: This research received no external funding.

Institutional Review Board Statement: Not applicable.

Informed Consent Statement: Not applicable.

Data Availability Statement: The data presented in this study are openly available at https://seer.cancer.gov/.

Conflicts of Interest: The authors declare no conflict of interest.

References

1. Scosyrev, E.; Noyes, K.; Feng, C.; Messing, E. Sex and racial differences in bladder cancer presentation and mortality in the US. *Cancer* **2009**, *115*, 68–74. [CrossRef] [PubMed]
2. Radkiewicz, C.; Edgren, G.; Johansson, A.L.V.; Jahnson, S.; Häggström, C.; Akre, O.; Lambe, M.; Dickman, P.W. Sex Differences in Urothelial Bladder Cancer Survival. *Clin. Genitourin. Cancer* **2020**, *18*, 26–34. [CrossRef] [PubMed]
3. Nakayama, M.; Ito, Y.; Hatano, K.; Nakai, Y.; Kakimoto, K.; Miyashiro, I.; Nishimura, K. Impact of sex difference on survival of bladder cancer: A population-based registry data in Japan. *Int. J. Urol.* **2019**, *26*, 649–654. [CrossRef]
4. Kluth, L.A.; Rieken, M.; Xylinas, E.; Kent, M.; Rink, M.; Rouprêt, M.; Sharifi, N.; Jamzadeh, A.; Kassouf, W.; Kaushik, D.; et al. Gender-specific differences in clinicopathologic outcomes following radical cystectomy: An international multi-institutional study of more than 8000 patients. *Eur Urol.* **2014**, *66*, 913. [CrossRef]
5. Otto, W.; May, M.; Fritsche, H.-M.; Dragun, D.; Aziz, A.; Gierth, M.; Trojan, L.; Herrmann, E.; Moritz, R.; Ellinger, J.; et al. Analysis of sex differences in cancer-specific survival and perioperative mortality following radical cystectomy: Results of a large german multicenter study of nearly 2500 patients with urothelial carcinoma of the bladder. *Gend. Med.* **2012**, *9*, 481–489. [CrossRef]
6. Tufano, A.; Cordua, N.; Nardone, V.; Ranavolo, R.; Flammia, R.S.; D'Antonio, F.; Borea, F.; Anceschi, U.; Leonardo, C.; Morrione, A.; et al. Prognostic Significance of Organ-Specific Metastases in Patients with Metastatic Upper Tract Urothelial Carcinoma. *J. Clin. Med.* **2022**, *11*, 5310. [CrossRef]

7. Messer, J.C.; Shariat, S.F.; Dinney, C.P.; Novara, G.; Fradet, Y.; Kassouf, W.; Karakiewicz, P.I.; Fritsche, H.-M.; Izawa, J.I.; Lotan, Y.; et al. Female gender is associated with a worse survival after radical cystectomy for urothelial carcinoma of the bladder: A competing risk analysis. *Urology* **2014**, *83*, 863–868. [CrossRef]
8. Rosiello, G.; Palumbo, C.; Pecoraro, A.; Luzzago, S.; Deuker, M.; Stolzenbach, L.F.; Tian, Z.; Gallina, A.; Gandaglia, G.; Montorsi, F.; et al. The effect of sex on disease stage and survival after radical cystectomy: A population-based analysis. *Urol. Oncol. Semin Orig. Investig.* **2021**, *39*, e1–e236. [CrossRef]
9. Uhlig, A.; Hosseini, A.S.A.; Simon, J.; Lotz, J.; Trojan, L.; Schmid, M.; Uhlig, J. Gender Specific Differences in Disease-Free, Cancer Specific and Overall Survival after Radical Cystectomy for Bladder Cancer: A Systematic Review and Meta-Analysis. *J. Urol.* **2018**, *200*, 48–60. [CrossRef]
10. Humphrey, P.A.; Moch, H.; Cubilla, A.L.; Ulbright, T.M.; Reuter, V.E. The 2016 WHO Classification of Tumours of the Urinary System and Male Genital Organs—Part B: Prostate and Bladder Tumours. *Eur. Urol.* **2016**, *70*, 106–119. [CrossRef] [PubMed]
11. Flammia, R.S.; Chierigo, F.; Würnschimmel, C.; Wenzel, M.; Horlemann, B.; Tian, Z.; Borghesi, M.; Leonardo, C.; Tilki, D.; Shariat, S.F.; et al. Sex-related differences in non-urothelial variant histology, non-muscle invasive bladder cancer. *Cent. Eur. J. Urol.* **2022**, *75*, 240–247. [CrossRef]
12. Deuker, M.; Martin, T.; Stolzenbach, F.; Rosiello, G.; Collà Ruvolo, C.; Karakiewicz, P.I. Bladder Cancer: A Comparison Between Non-urothelial Variant Histology and Urothelial Carcinoma Across All Stages and Treatment Modalities. *Clin. Genitourin. Cancer* **2021**, *19*, 60–68.e1. [CrossRef]
13. Flaig, T.W.; Spiess, P.E.; Agarwal, N.; Bangs, R.; Boorjian, S.A.; Buyyounouski, M.K.; Chang, S.; Downs, T.M.; Efstathiou, J.A.; Friedlander, T.; et al. Bladder Cancer, Version 3.2020, NCCN Clinical Practice Guidelines in Oncology. *J. Natl. Compr Cancer Netw* **2020**, *18*, 329–354. [CrossRef]
14. Pottegård, A.; Kristensen, K.B.; Friis, S.; Hallas, J.; Jensen, J.B.; Nørgaard, M. Urinary tract infections and risk of squamous cell carcinoma bladder cancer: A Danish nationwide case-control study. *Int. J. Cancer* **2020**, *146*, 1930–1936. [CrossRef]
15. Noon, A.; Albertsen, P.C.; Thomas, F.; Rosario, D.J.; Catto, J.W.F. Competing mortality in patients diagnosed with bladder cancer: Evidence of undertreatment in the elderly and female patients. *Br. J. Cancer* **2013**, *108*, 1534–1540. [CrossRef]
16. Månsson, Å.; Anderson, H.; Colleen, S. Time lag to diagnosis of bladder cancer-influence of psychosocial parameters and level of health-care provision. *Scand. J. Urol. Nephrol.* **1993**, *27*, 363–369. [CrossRef]
17. Ark, J.T.; Alvarez, J.R.; Koyama, T.; Bassett, J.C.; Blot, W.J.; Mumma, M.T.; Resnick, M.J.; You, C.; Penson, D.; Barocas, D.A. Variation in the Diagnostic Evaluation among Persons with Hematuria: Influence of Gender, Race and Risk Factors for Bladder Cancer. *J. Urol.* **2017**, *198*, 1033–1038. [CrossRef]
18. Cohn, J.A.; Vekhter, B.; Lyttle, C.; Steinberg, G.D.; Large, M.C. Sex disparities in diagnosis of bladder cancer after initial resentation with hematuria: A nationwide claims-based investigation. *Cancer* **2014**, *120*, 555–561. [CrossRef]
19. Santos, F.; Dragomir, A.; Kassouf, W.; Franco, E.; Aprikian, A. Urologist referral delay and its impact on survival after radical cystectomy for bladder cancer. *Curr. Oncol.* **2015**, *22*, 20–26. [CrossRef]
20. Barocas, D.A.; Boorjian, S.A.; Alvarez, R.D.; Downs, T.M.; Gross, C.P.; Hamilton, B.D.; Kobashi, K.C.; Lipman, R.R.; Lotan, Y.; Ng, C.K.; et al. Microhematuria: AUA/SUFU Guideline. *J. Urol.* **2020**, *204*, 778–786. [CrossRef]
21. Woldu, S.L.; Ng, C.K.; Loo, R.K.; Slezak, J.M.; Jacobsen, S.J.; Tan, W.S.; Kelly, J.D.; Lough, T.; Darling, D.; van Kessel, K.E.M. et al. Evaluation of the New American Urological Association Guidelines Risk Classification for Hematuria. *J. Urol.* **2021**, *205*, 1387–1393. [CrossRef] [PubMed]
22. Mir, C.; Shariat, S.F.; Van der Kwast, T.; Ashfaq, R.; Lotan, Y.; Evans, A.; Skeldon, S.; Hanna, S.; Vajpeyi, R.; Kuk, C.; et al. Loss of androgen receptor expression is not associated with pathological stage, grade, gender or outcome in bladder cancer: A large multi-institutional study. *BJU Int.* **2011**, *108*, 24–30. [CrossRef] [PubMed]
23. Del Giudice, F.; Busetto, G.M.; Gross, M.S.; Maggi, M.; Sciarra, A.; Salciccia, S.; Ferro, M.; Sperduti, I.; Flammia, S.; Canale, V.; et al. Efficacy of three BCG strains (Connaught, TICE and RIVM) with or without secondary resection (re-TUR) for intermediate/high risk non-muscle-invasive bladder cancers: Results from a retrospective single-institution cohort analysis. *J. Cancer Res. Clin Oncol.* **2021**, *147*, 3073–3080. [CrossRef]
24. Sorce, G.; Chierigo, F.; Flammia, R.S.; Hoeh, B.; Hohenhorst, L.; Tian, Z.; Goyal, J.A.; Graefen, M.; Terrone, C.; Gallucci, M.; et al. Survival trends in chemotherapy exposed metastatic bladder cancer patients and chemotherapy effect across different age, sex and race/ethnicity. *Urol. Oncol.* **2022**, *40*, e19–e380. [CrossRef] [PubMed]
25. Flammia, R.S.; Chierigo, F.; Würnschimmel, C.; Horlemann, B.; Gallucci, M.; Karakiewicz, P.I. Survival benefit of chemotherapy in a contemporary cohort of metastatic urachal carcinoma. *Urol. Oncol.* **2022**, *40*, 165.e9–165.e15. [CrossRef]
26. Sorce, G.; Flammia, R.S.; Hoeh, B.; Chierigo, F.; Briganti, A.; Karakiewicz, P.I. Plasmacytoid variant urothelial carcinoma of the bladder: Effect of radical cystectomy and chemotherapy in non-metastatic and metastatic patients. *World J. Urol.* **2022**, *40*, 1481–1488. [CrossRef] [PubMed]

Disclaimer/Publisher's Note: The statements, opinions and data contained in all publications are solely those of the individual author(s) and contributor(s) and not of MDPI and/or the editor(s). MDPI and/or the editor(s) disclaim responsibility for any injury to people or property resulting from any ideas, methods, instructions or products referred to in the content.

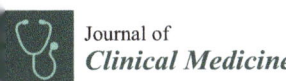

Article

Diminishing the Gender-Related Disparity in Survival among Chemotherapy Pre-Treated Patients after Radical Cystectomy—A Multicenter Observational Study

Krystian Kaczmarek [1,*], Artur Lemiński [1], Bartosz Małkiewicz [2], Adam Gurwin [2], Janusz Lisiński [1] and Marcin Słojewski [1]

1 Department of Urology and Urological Oncology, Pomeranian Medical University, Powstańców Wielkopolskich 72, 70-111 Szczecin, Poland
2 Department of Minimally Invasive and Robotic Urology, University Center of Excellence in Urology, Wrocław Medical University, Borowska 213, 50-556 Wrocław, Poland
* Correspondence: k.kaczmarek.md@gmail.com; Tel.: +48-91-4661100

Abstract: There is a well-documented problem of inferior outcome of muscle-invasive bladder cancer (MIBC) after radical cystectomy (RC) in women. However, previous studies were conducted before neoadjuvant chemotherapy (NAC) was widely adopted to multidisciplinary management of MIBC. In our study, we assessed the gender-related difference in survival between patients who received NAC and those who underwent upfront RC, in two academic centers. This non-randomized, clinical follow-up study enrolled 1238 consecutive patients, out of whom 253 received NAC. We analyzed survival outcome of RC according to gender between NAC and non-NAC subgroups. We found that female gender was associated with inferior overall survival (OS), compared to males (HR, 1.234; 95%CI 1.046–1.447; $p = 0.013$) in the overall cohort and in non-NAC patients with $\geq$pT2 disease (HR, 1.220 95%CI 1.009–1.477; $p = 0.041$). However, no gender-specific difference was observed in patients exposed to NAC. The 5-year OS in NAC-exposed women in $\leq$pT1 and $\geq$pT2 disease, was 69.333% 95%CI (46.401–92.265) and 36.535% (13.134–59.936) respectively, compared to men 77.727% 95%CI (65.952–89.502) and 39.122% 95%CI (29.162–49.082), respectively. The receipt of NAC not only provides downstaging and prolongs patients' survival after radical treatment of MIBC but may also help to diminish the gender specific disparity.

Keywords: bladder cancer; gender disparity; neoadjuvant therapy; radical cystectomy

1. Introduction

According to population-based studies, women have better survival rates, compared to men, after diagnosis of most cancers [1]. However, no such phenomenon is observed in bladder cancer (BC). The risk of BC progression and mortality is higher in women than in men [2]. In contrast, men are more likely to develop BC than women [1]. This gap in oncological outcomes may be partially attributed to more advanced stage at presentation in women [3]. The initially higher T-stage is mainly explained by a longer delay in the diagnosis of BC in women than in men, whereby a urinary tract infection (UTI) might be regarded as the culprit of a misdiagnosis of BC due to association with hematuria and higher prevalence among women. Although UTIs are more common in women <40 years old, a limited assessment of a gross hematuria is still seen in older women [4]. The gender-related survival disparity is also observed in stage-to-stage comparisons between women and men and is particularly pronounced in advanced stages of BC; hence, higher presenting stage in women cannot fully clarify this phenomenon [3]. Moreover, differences in gender-specific survival persist after radical cystectomy (RC). This emphasizes the complexity of this issue and the potential impact of other factors, such as treatment availability and patterns, tobacco smoking, chemical exposure, and hormonal status [5]. An association of gender with long-term outcomes of RC has been extensively analyzed before the widespread adoption of neoadjuvant chemotherapy (NAC) [6,7]. Administration of NAC is the current standard of care for patients with muscle-invasive bladder cancer (MIBC) eligible for cisplatin therapy and provides up to 50% of downstaging to <ypT2N0, with complete remissions achievable in one-third of patients [8,9]. Moreover, NAC improves overall survival (OS) by 5–8% at 5 years, equivalent to a number needed to treat of 12.5 [10]. Besides NAC, currently there is an increasing number of promising precisely targeted agents which are assessing for use in neoadjuvant setting in BC. These agents might be use alone or in combination with traditional chemotherapy [11]. However, cisplatin-based combination chemotherapy remains a recommended treatment before RC. Nevertheless, data regarding the gender inequality in survival after RC in the NAC era are limited. Therefore, in this evolving landscape of treatment for MIBC, we decided to conduct a study which answers a question of whether the gender-related disparity in survival in patients undergoing upfront RC would still be observed after exposure to NAC.

In the present study, we hypothesized that the administration of NAC not only improves mid-term outcome after RC, but may as well diminish the survival disadvantage among women after RC. Hence, the objective of our study was to reassess the differences in gender-specific survival between chemotherapy pre-treated and chemotherapy-naïve patients undergoing RC in the NAC era.

2. Material and Methods

This non-randomized clinical follow-up study was exempt from further review by the Institutional Review Board (Bioethical Committee) of the Pomeranian Medical University, Szczecin, Poland (protocol number KB. 006.102.2022/Z-9521) and was conducted according to the regulations set forth by the Declaration of Helsinki. Consent for research participation was routinely obtained from all patients involved, namely, for the use of their anonymized treatment data collected during hospitalization. Consecutive patients who underwent RC and pelvic lymphadenectomy due to MIBC at two university centers—the Department of Urology and Urological Oncology of the Pomeranian Medical University, Szczecin, Poland, and the Department of Minimally Invasive and Robotic Urology, University Center of Excellence in Urology of Wroclaw Medical University, Poland—were enrolled in the study. Patients were treated between 1991–2021 and 2003–2021, in first and second participating department, respectively. Patients with metastatic disease, those who underwent cystectomy for palliative indications, those who underwent partial bladder resections, patients with a history of pelvic radiotherapy, and those with non-urothelial pathology were excluded from analysis. In total, 99 patients were excluded, and the data of 1238 patients were utilized for statistical analyses. The analyzed cohort was divided into two groups according to NAC administration. NAC was administered to 253 patients until the end of 2021. The remaining study population underwent upfront RC with eventual adjuvant treatment depending on the final pathologic stage (non-NAC group, n = 985). The NAC cisplatin-based chemotherapy was offered patients who meet all eligibility criteria, including Eastern Cooperative Oncology Group Performance Status (ECOG PS) 0–1, glomerular filtration rate (GFR) > 60 mL/min, audiometric hearing loss grade < 2, peripheral neuropathy grade < 2, and function of the heart according to the New York Heart Association Functional Classification < III. If patent did not fulfill all those criteria and ECOG PS was at least 2 and GFR was between 30–60 mL/min, then carboplatin-based chemotherapy was considered. However, if GFR was <60 mL/min and ECOG PS < 2 and the patient had adequate bone marrow reserve, then taxane-based chemotherapy was offered after individual assessment by oncological team. No patient was exposed to immuno-oncology therapy before RC. To identify differences between genders, we evaluated the association between gender and long-term oncological outcome in both groups according to the pathological stage (Figure 1). Data were reviewed for internal consistency. Descriptive statistics including mean ± standard deviation (SD) and median (interquartile range, IQR) were applied for normally distributed and skewed data, respectively. Single variables were compared using an independent t-test (parametric variables) and a chi-square test (non-parametric variables). If the Cochran's assumptions for chi-square test were not met, the Fisher–Freeman–Halton test was applied. OS probabilities over time were presented using Kaplan–Meier survival estimates and univariate Cox models. The survival curves of different groups were compared using the log-rank test. Multivariable Cox proportional hazard models were applied to examine the impact of prognostic factors on survival, including age at the time of surgery, gender, the severity of comorbidities reflected by the American Society of Anesthesiologists (ASA) score, pathological T stage, cancer grade, and pathological lymph node status. To test for independence between residuals and time, an assessment of the proportional hazard assumption of final multivariable models was performed using scaled Schoenfeld residuals with time. The results of Cox proportional hazard models were presented as hazard ratios (HR) with their 95% confidence intervals (CIs). Additionally, because patients were not randomly assigned to administration of NAC, we performed propensity scores analyses. Logistic regression was used to calculate propensity scores to estimate the predictive probabilities of receiving NAC. We considered p value < 0.05 as statistically significant and all p values were two-sided. All tests were performed using Statistica software, version 13.5 (StatSoft, Inc., Tulsa, OK, USA) and R (version 4.2.2) and RStudio (version 2022.12.0) with R packages *survival*, *survminer*, *drylr*.

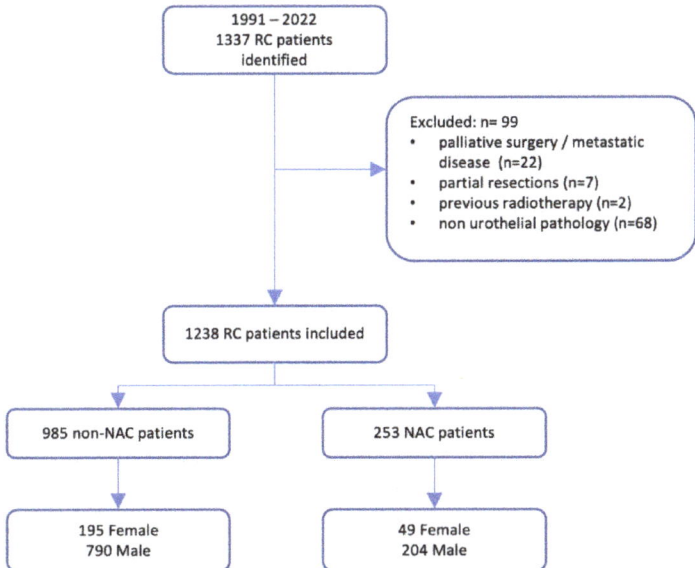

Figure 1. Flowchart of the study. NAC: neoadjuvant chemotherapy; RC: radical cystectomy.

3. Results

Out of 1238 patients included in the study, 253 (20.4%) received NAC. The median follow-up time was 23.467 months (IQR, 8.800–52.233), and there were no significant differences between genders (women, 21.333 months [IQR, 8.783–50.667] vs. men, 23.967 months [IQR, 8.800–52.233]). Women were generally older at the time of surgery and had higher pathological cancer stage than men. Statistically, greater proportion of women had extravesical disease (65.98% and 57.14% respectively; $p = 0.007$). However, there were no significant differences in lymph node metastasis, tumor grade, and ASA score distributions (Table 1).

Table 1. Baseline patients' characteristics according to gender.

Variable	Female	Male	p Value
Totals, No. (%)	244 (19.71)	994 (80.29)	
Age, years			0.006
Mean	66.709	64.79	
SD	9.88	8.64	
ASA score, No. (%)			0.082
1	17 (6.97)	99 (9.96)	
2	169 (69.26)	611 (61.47)	
3	58 (23.77)	277 (27.87)	
4	0 (0.00)	7 (0.70)	
Pathological T stage, No. (%)			0.007
pT0	23 (9.43)	80 (8.05)	
pTis/Ta/T1	22 (9.02)	153 (15.39)	
pT2	38 (15.57)	193 (19.42)	
pT3	95 (38.93)	288 (28.97)	
pT4	66 (27.05)	280 (28.17)	
Pathological N stage, No. (%)			0.319
pN0	151 (61.89)	649 (65.29)	
pN+	93 (38.11)	345 (34.71)	
Cancer grade, No. (%)			0.213
Low grade	12 (4.92)	71 (7.14)	
High grade	232 (95.08)	923 (92.86)	
Neoadjuvant chemotherapy, No. (%)			0.878
No	195 (79.92)	790 (79.48)	
Yes	49 (20.08)	204 (20.52)	
Chemotherapy regimen, No. (%)			0.515
ddMVAC	21 (8.61)	96 (9.66)	
Gemcitabine-cisplatin	27 (11.07)	92 (9.26)	
Gemcitabine-carboplatin	0 (0.00)	5 (0.50)	
Gemcitabine-paclitaxel	1 (0.41)	11 (1.11)	
Cycles of chemotherapy, No, (%)			0.894
<3	19 (7.79)	77 (7.75)	
≥3	30 (12.30)	127 (12.78)	
Department, No. (%)			0.044
Szczecin	117 (47.95)	406 (40.85)	
Wrocław	127 (52.05)	588 (59.15)	
Follow-up, months			0.746
media	21.333	23.967	
IQ	8.783–50.667	8.800–52.233	

ASA score: American Society of Anesthesiologists score; IQR: interquartile range; SD standard deviation.

No significant difference between women and men was found regarding exposure to NAC (women 20.08% vs. men 20.52%), chemotherapy regimen, and number of NAC cycles administered (Table 1). NAC provided disease downstaging to <ypT2N0 in 86 (33.99%) patients, including complete responses (CR) in 43 (17.00%; Table 2). No significant differences between women and men were observed in response rates to NAC. Complete remissions were observed in 22.45% of women and 14.71% of men ($p = 0.187$), whereas partial responses (<ypT2N0) were noted in 34.69% of women and 30.39% of men ($p = 0.560$). However, there were significant differences in response to NAC between participating centers. In the Department of Urology and Urological Oncology in Szczecin, CR was achieved in 22% of patients, whereas the rate of complete remissions in the Department of Minimally Invasive and Robotic Urology in Wrocław reached only 12% ($p = 0.043$). Correspondingly, significant difference was observed in partial response rates (40.0% and 25.49% respectively, $p = 0.015$). Further heterogeneity was observed regarding preferred cytotoxic regimens. In Szczecin, 59 (59%) patients received dose-dense methotrexate vinblastine, doxorubicin, and cisplatin (ddMVAC) regimen, as compared to 58 (37.9%) patients who were exposed to NAC in Wrocław ($p < 0.001$). Furthermore, fewer patients received an optimal number of NAC cycles (≥3) in Wroclaw, as compared to Szczecin (55.6% versus 72.0%, $p = 0.008$).

Table 2. Baseline patients' characteristics according to expose to neoadjuvant chemotherapy.

Variable	non-NAC	NAC	p Value
Totals, No. (%)	985 (79.56)	253 (20.44)	
Age, years			0.431
Mean	65.27	64.77	
SD	9.13	8.11	
Gender, No. (%)			0.878
Female	195 (19.80)	49 (19.37)	
Male	790 (80.20)	204 (80.63)	
ASA score, No. (%)			0.084
1	96 (9.75)	20 (7.91)	
2	633 (64.26)	147 (58.10)	
3	251 (25.48)	84 (33.20)	
4	5 (0.51)	2 (0.79)	
Pathological T stage, No. (%)			<0.001
pT0	60 (6.09)	43 (17.00)	
pTis/Ta/T1	132 (13.40)	43 (17.00)	
pT2	177 (17.97)	54 (21.34)	
pT3	330 (33.50)	53 (20.95)	
pT4	286 (29.04)	60 (23.72)	
Pathological N stage, No. (%)			0.161
pN0	627 (63.65)	173 (68.38)	
pN+	358 (36.35)	80 (31.62)	
Cancer grade, No. (%)			<0.001
Low grade	81 (8.22)	2 (0.79)	
High grade	904 (91.78)	241 (99.21)	
Chemotherapy regimen, No. (%)			
ddMVAC	n/a	117 (9.44)	
Gemcitabine-cisplatin	n/a	119 (9.60)	
Gemcitabine-carboplatin	n/a	5 (0.40)	
Gemcitabine-paclitaxel	n/a	12 (0.97)	
Cycles of chemotherapy, No, (%)			
<3	n/a	96 (7.75)	
≥3	n/a	157 (12.68)	
Department, No. (%)			0.326
Szczecin	423 (42.94)	100 (39.53)	
Wrocław	562 (57.06)	153 (60.47)	
Follow-up, months			0.155
median	21.77	29.40	
IQR	8.00–53.27	10.43–49.57	

ASA score: American Society of Anesthesiologists score; IQR: interquartile range; SD standard deviation.

Kaplan–Meier survival curves and Cox regression analyses were performed in the entire cohort and revealed that OS observed in women was inferior to that in men (HR, 1.234; 95% CI, 1.046–1.447; $p = 0.013$). The 5-year OS for women and men was 32.906% (95% CI, 26.215–39.597) and 41.819% (95% CI, 38.377–45.261), respectively. After stratification by pT stage, inferior OS was observed in women with ≥pT2 disease, as compared to men (HR, 1.218; 95%CI, 1.017–1.458; $p = 0.032$). The 5-year OS for women and men with ≥pT2 disease was 24.926% (95% CI, 18.267–31.585) and 32.596% (95% CI, 28.821–36.371), respectively. The difference was consistently observed in a subset of patients with ≥pT2 disease who did not receive NAC, with a 5-year OS of 25.511% (95% CI, 18.688–32.334) in women as opposed to 32.596% (95% CI, 28.821–36.371) in men (HR, 1.220; 95%CI, 1.009–1.477; $p = 0.041$). However, no gender-specific difference was observed across stage groups in patients who received NAC. The 5-year OS in the NAC group for women in ≤ypT1 and ≥ypT2 disease was 69.333% (95% CI, 46.401–92.265) and 36.535% (95% CI, 13.134–59.936), respectively as opposed to 77.727% (95% CI, 65.952–89.502) and 39.122% (95% CI, 29.162–49.082), in men (Figure 2). These findings were validated using a competing risk regression model. In multivariable analysis, the difference in OS was observed in the non-NAC ≥pT2 group (HR, 1.229; 95%CI, 1.013–1.492; p = 0.036). However, administration of NAC diminished gender-specific disparities in OS after RC also among patients who did not respond to neoadjuvant therapy (HR, 1.136; 95%CI, 0.630–2.046; p = 0.672; Table 3; Table S1). These results were confirmed in propensity scores analysis (Table S2).

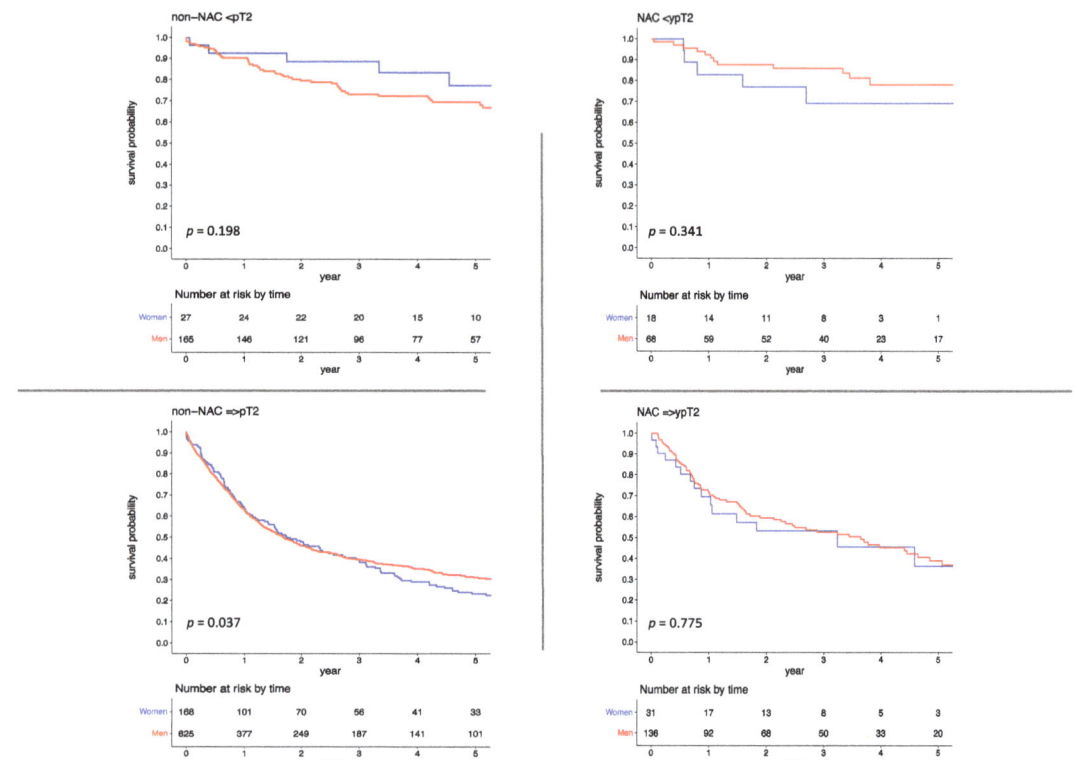

Figure 2. Kaplan–Meier analysis of overall survival in chemotherapy-naïve and chemotherapy pre-treated patients who underwent radical cystectomy stratified according to tumor stage.

Table 3. Impact of female sex on overall survival in univariable, multivariable and propensity-weighted regression analysis stratified by pT stage and receipt of neoadjuvant chemotherapy.

		UNIVARIABLE				MULTIVARIABLE *				PROPENSITY SCORE **		
	HR	Lower CI	Upper CI	p	HR	Lower CI	Upper CI	p	HR	Lower CI	Upper CI	p
					All patients							
all	1.234	1.046	1.447	0.013	1.103	0.926	1.314	0.271	1.171	0.974	1.408	0.093
<pT2	0.830	0.440	1.567	0.566	0.844	0.430	1.659	0.624	0.777	0.401	1.505	0.454
≥pT2	1.218	1.017	1.458	0.032	1.219	1.015	1.463	0.034	1.226	1.011	1.486	0.038
					non-NAC							
all	1.244	1.034	1.496	0.021	1.162	0.963	1.402	0.118	1.168	0.958	1.425	0.125
<pT2	0.584	0.252	1.353	0.210	0.726	0.314	1.680	0.454	0.555	0.232	1.331	0.187
≥pT2	1.220	1.009	1.477	0.041	1.229	1.013	1.492	0.036	1.241	1.011	1.524	0.039

Table 3. Cont.

	UNIVARIABLE				MULTIVARIABLE *				PROPENSITY SCORE **			
	HR	Lower CI	Upper CI	p	HR	Lower CI	Upper CI	p	HR	Lower CI	Upper CI	p
					NAC							
all	1.151	0.706	1.877	0.572	1.228	0.732	2.059	0.437	1.228	0.732	2.059	0.437
<ypT2	1.683	0.596	4.748	0.325	1.852	0.603	5.690	0.282	1.852	0.603	5.690	0.282
≥ypT2	1.090	0.624	1.904	0.762	1.136	0.630	2.046	0.672	1.136	0.630	2.046	0.672

* Adjusted for age, gender, severity of comorbidities reflected by American Society of Anesthesiologists, pathological T stage, pathological N stage, tumor grade, neoadjuvant chemotherapy. ** Weighted for age, gender, severity of comorbidities reflected by American Society of Anesthesiologists. CI: confidenceinterval; HR: hazard ratio; NAC: neoadjuvant chemotherapy.

4. Discussion

Gender-related survival differences in BC are well documented and more pronounced among patients undergoing RC [5,12–14]. These findings are surprising given that women generally have better disease-specific survival than men for most cancers affecting both sexes [15–17]. This phenomenon has not been fully elucidated, with current hypotheses including longer delay from presentation with hematuria to diagnosis in women, anatomic and hormonal differences, higher stage at presentation, and variation in tumor biology [4,11,18–20]. However, once diagnosed with MIBC, data on sex-specific responses to different treatment regimens and the influence on oncological outcomes is limited.

In our study, women undergoing RC due to MIBC showed inferior OS when compared with men, which is in line with previous reports [5,14]. However, the difference in our cohort was more significant. The HR in the overall cohort was 1.234 (95% CI, 1.046–1.447). According to Krimphove et al., who used data from the National Cancer Database, women presenting with MIBC accounted for only 4% and were slightly more likely to die than men (HR, 1.04; 95% CI, 1.00–1.07) [21]. The difference was even less pronounced in other studies [2,22]. Variations in observed outcomes between the studies may be attributed to the differences in sample size, period of treatment, and study design. Our cohort was more homogeneous than cohorts in previous studies as we excluded patients with pathological variants of BC other than urothelial carcinoma and included patients who underwent RC at academic centers. Moreover, the differences between gender may be related to the increasing prevalence of tobacco-related BC among women in Poland. The highest exposure to smoking, which reached 50%, was reported in generation of Polish women born between 1940 and 1960 [23]. Therefore, considering the latency time and cohort effect, the incidence and mortality due to BC in women showed an increasing trend, which may explain the higher disproportion in OS observed between genders in our study.

In the subgroup analysis of patients with ≥pT2 disease sex-related differences observed for all cohort persisted, with unadjusted and adjusted HR of 1.218 (95% CI, 1.017–1.458) and 1.219 (95% CI, 1.015–1.463), respectively. After further stratification of this group according to NAC exposure, the survival gap was evident in chemotherapy-naïve patients (HR, 1.229; 95% CI, 1.013–1.492), but was no longer found in patients who received NAC, in whom OS of women was comparable to that of men (HR, 1.136; 95% CI, 0.630–2.046). Equivalent results were presented in meta-analysis by Kimura et al. who analyzed the association between gender and oncologic outcomes in the NAC pretreated cohort. In their study, gender was not associated with overall mortality. Similarly, no correlation with CR or partial response was found. Of note, women undergoing NAC and RC were less likely to have tumor upstaging at the time of surgery than men [24].

Diminishment of gender-related OS gap in NAC pre-treated patients after RC may be partially explained at molecular level. According to the Cancer Genome Atlas, MIBC is divided into two main subgroups: luminal and basal-squamous. Each type is associated with distinct histopathological features, prognosis, and treatment implications [25]. Robertson et al. discovered that BC in women was mostly categorized as the basal-squamous subtype, which expressed high levels of CTLA4 and CD274 (PD-L1) immunomarkers and responded well to immune therapy [26]. Moreover, Seiler et al. highlighted that this molecular subtype showed greater response rate and survival improvement after NAC-RC, compared to other subtypes and cystectomy alone. Given higher proportion of basal-squamous subtype in women, we hypothesize NAC may yield better responses in female patients [27].

Another potential reason for comparable survival outcomes observed between sexes after NAC exposure may be related to difference in bladder wall thickness. The bladder wall is thinner in women than in men, which may facilitate more thorough transurethral resection of bladder tumor (TURBT) [28]. James et al. showed the association between maximal TURBT and improved survival and oncologic outcomes in a cohort of patients with MIBC. NAC pretreated patients who underwent maximal TURBT were more likely to achieve a complete pathologic response (odds ratio 3.17; 95% CI, 1.02–9.83) [29]. Similar results were reported by other authors [30].

Several NAC regimens were analyzed in this study. A significant proportion of patients were treated with ddMVAC regimen (46.25%), which may have affected our results. Haines et al. analyzed the association between gender and outcomes in patients with metastatic urothelial carcinoma and revealed a significantly longer survival in women than in men treated with MVAC (methotrexate, vinblastine, doxorubicin, and cisplatin), whereas no gender-related differences were observed in patients treated with gemcitabine and cisplatin regimens. However, these findings should be interpreted with caution given the small sample size of female patients treated with MVAC [31]. Therefore, an improved female response to ddMVAC is a hypothesis rather than a firm conclusion [9]. However gender-related differences in response to particular regimens are not implausible.

Our present study has limitations, and the results should be interpreted within the limitations of the observational study design. Firstly, we were unable to analyze unmeasured confounding factors, such as socioeconomic status, comorbidities using the Charlson Comorbidity Index, smoking status, clinical stage, and adjuvant chemotherapy, which may have influenced survival. Hence, we also could not have provided a rate of clinical understaging in patients who underwent upfront RC. Secondly, there were significant disparities between participating centers regarding chemotherapy regimens, number of administered cycles, and response to neoadjuvant treatment. A plausible explanation of this phenomenon may include different treatment periods. Patients from the Department of Urology in Szczecin were treated more recently, when the role of NAC in the treatment of MIBC was firmly established, whereas in Wroclaw, the analysis, spanning over a period of 30 years, included the early era of NAC [32]. This discrepancy may be one of reasons why more patients in Wroclaw received less optimal regimens. Thirdly, as data regarding cause of death was not always available, our survival analysis was limited to OS, which may have introduced additional bias due to concurrent mortality, potentially significant in this population. Lastly, we are aware that currently there are ongoing studies, investigating novel therapeutic opportunities in neoadjuvant setting in MIBC. Preliminary results of these trials suggested that using agents such as checkpoint inhibitors before RC has clear potential advantages, due to their acceptable tolerance and high efficacy. Hence, soon, we might see changes in the landscape of treatment of BC [33,34]. Moreover, currently observing gender-related disparities among patients who are not exposing to neoadjuvant therapy might not be observed as more patients will be eligible to multidisciplinary approach. Thus only palliative cases will be treated with upfront cystectomy.

Despite these limitations, we believe that this study provides a reliable analysis of gender-specific outcomes of early multidisciplinary management of MIBC. One of the strengths of the present study is the novelty of results addressing diminishing gender specific disparities in survival in patients regardless of response status to NAC. In previous reports addressing sex-specific disparities after NAC administration, a reduction of survival gap was only observed in patients with pT4 disease [35,36]. Our results highlighted that women who have no pathological response to NAC may benefit from multidisciplinary treatment. Administration of NAC may help to mediate influence of potential sex-related factors, such as delayed diagnosis, anatomical differences, higher stage at the time of diagnosis, or altered tumor biology, which likely contribute to differences in oncologic outcomes.

5. Conclusions

In summary, our results highlight that the administration of neoadjuvant chemotherapy helps decrease the gender-related survival gap after radical cystectomy. Thus, we believe that female patients may benefit from gender-specific counseling regarding perioperative therapeutic strategies and personalized medicine approaches to greater extent than male patients. However, lack of gender-associated disparities in the survival of patients with muscle invasive bladder cancer after multidisciplinary treatment cannot be entirely proven based on the limitations of the study and further large, prospective studies are needed. Furthermore, in the light of an ongoing era of immunotherapy in advanced bladder cancer, the gender-related disparities should be studied simultaneously with the efficacy of new agents.

Supplementary Materials: The following supporting information can be downloaded at: https://www.mdpi.com/article/10.3390/jcm12041260/s1, Table S1: Multivariable regression analysis of factors predicting overall survival. Available at: https://osf.io/kr4w6. Table S2: Multivariable propensity-weighted regression analysis of factors predicting overall survival. Available at: https://osf.io/kqbgr.

Author Contributions: Conceptualization, K.K. and A.L.; methodology, K.K.; formal analysis, K.K. and A.L.; investigation, K.K. and A.L.; data curation, K.K., A.L., B.M., J.L. and A.G.; writing—original draft preparation, K.K. and A.L.; writing—review and editing, K.K. and A.L.; visualization, K.K.; supervision, M.S.; project administration, K.K., A.L., B.M. and M.S. All authors have read and agreed to the published version of the manuscript.

Funding: This research received no external funding.

Institutional Review Board Statement: The study was conducted in accordance with the Declaration of Helsinki and approved by the Institutional Review Board (Bioethical Committee) of the Pomeranian Medical University, Szczecin, Poland (protocol number KB. 006.102.2022/Z-9521).

Informed Consent Statement: Subjects involved were routinely consented for scientific use of anonymized treatment data at the time of hospital stay.

Data Availability Statement: Source data available at: https://osf.io/bsnt5.

Acknowledgments: The authors would like to thank Barbara Zawisza-Lemińska and Marta Wiącek for their continuous support and contribution.

Conflicts of Interest: The authors declare no conflict of interest.

References

1. Siegel, R.L.; Miller, K.D.; Fuchs, H.E.; Jemal ASiegel, R.L.; Miller, K.D.; Fuchs, H.E.; Jemal, A. Cancer Statistics, 2021. *CA Cancer J. Clin.* **2021**, *71*, 7–33. [CrossRef] [PubMed]
2. Uhlig, A.; Hosseini, A.S.A.; Simon, J.; Lotz, J.; Trojan, L.; Schmid, M.; Uhlig, J. Gender Specific Differences in Disease-Free, Cancer Specific and Overall Survival after Radical Cystectomy for Bladder Cancer: A Systematic Review and Meta-Analysis. *J. Urol.* **2018**, *200*, 48–60. [CrossRef]
3. Waldhoer, T.; Berger, I.; Haidinger, G.; Zielonke, N.; Madersbacher SWaldhoer, T.; Berger, I.; Haidinger, G.; Zielonke, N.; Madersbacher, S. Sex differences of ≥pT1 bladder cancer survival in Austria: A descriptive, long-term, na-tion-wide analysis based on 27,773 patients. *Urol Int.* **2015**, *94*, 383–389. [CrossRef]
4. Johnson, E.K.; Daignault, S.; Zhang, Y.; Lee CTJohnson, E.K.; Daignault, S.; Zhang, Y.; Lee, C.T. Patterns of Hematuria Referral to Urologists: Does a Gender Disparity Exist? *Urology* **2008**, *72*, 498–502. [CrossRef] [PubMed]
5. Dobruch, J.; Daneshmand, S.; Fisch, M.; Lotan, Y.; Noon, A.P.; Resnick, M.J.; Shariat, S.F.; Zlotta, A.R.; Boorjian, S.A. Gender and Bladder Cancer: A Collaborative Review of Etiology, Biology, and Outcomes. *Eur. Urol.* **2016**, *69*, 300–310. [CrossRef]
6. Soave, A.; Dahlem, R.; Hansen, J.; Weisbach, L.; Minner, S.; Engel, O.; Kluth, L.; Chun, F.; Shariat, S.; Fisch, M.; et al. Gender-specific outcomes of bladder cancer patients: A stage-specific analysis in a contemporary, homogenous radical cystectomy cohort. *Eur. J. Surg. Oncol. (EJSO)* **2014**, *41*, 368–377. [CrossRef] [PubMed]

7. Liu, S.; Yang, T.; Na, R.; Hu, M.; Zhang, L.; Fu, Y.; Jiang, H.; Ding, Q. The impact of female gender on bladder cancer-specific death risk after radical cystectomy: A meta-analysis of 27,912 patients. *Int. Urol. Nephrol.* **2015**, *47*, 951–958. [CrossRef]
8. Peyton, C.C.; Tang, D.; Reich, R.R.; Azizi, M.; Chipollini, J.; Pow-Sang, J.M.; Manley, B.; Spiess, P.E.; Poch, M.A.; Sexton, W.J.; et al. Downstaging and Survival Outcomes Associated with Neoadjuvant Chemo-therapy Regimens among Patients Treated with Cystectomy for Muscle-Invasive Bladder Cancer Supplemental content. *JAMA Oncol.* **2018**, *4*, 1535–1542. [CrossRef]
9. Lemiński, A.; Kaczmarek, K.; Byrski, T.; Słojewski, M. Neoadjuvant chemotherapy with dose dense MVAC is associated with improved survival after radical cystectomy compared to other cytotoxic regimens: A tertiary center experience. *PLoS ONE* **2021**, *16*, e0259526. [CrossRef]
10. Yin, M.; Joshi, M.; Meijer, R.P.; Glantz, M.; Holder, S.; Harvey, H.A.; Kaag, M.; Fransen van de Putte, E.E.; Horenblas, S.; Drabick, J.J. Neoadjuvant Chemotherapy for Muscle-Invasive Bladder Cancer: A Systematic Re-view and Two-Step Meta-Analysis. *Oncologist* **2016**, *21*, 708–715. [CrossRef]
11. Cheetham, P.J.; Petrylak, D.P. New Agents for the Treatment of Advanced Bladder Cancer. *Oncology* **2016**, *30*, 571–579, 588.
12. Mallin, K.; David, K.A.; Carroll, P.R.; Milowsky, M.I.; Nanus, D.M. Transitional Cell Carcinoma of the Bladder: Racial and Gender Disparities in Survival (1993 to 2002), Stage and Grade (1993 to 2007). *J. Urol.* **2011**, *185*, 1631–1636. [CrossRef]
13. Boffa, D.J.; Rosen, J.E.; Mallin, K.; Loomis, A.; Gay, G.; Palis, B.; Thoburn, K.; Gress, D.; McKellar, D.P.; Shulman, L.N.; et al. Using the National Cancer Database for Outcomes Research: A Review. *JAMA Oncol.* **2017**, *3*, 1722–1728. [CrossRef]
14. Kluth, L.A.; Rieken, M.; Xylinas, E.; Kent, M.; Rink, M.; Rouprêt, M.; Sharifi, N.; Jamzadeh, A.; Kassouf, W.; Kaushik, D.; et al. Gender-specific Differences in Clinicopathologic Outcomes Following Radical Cystec-tomy: An International Multi-institutional Study of More Than 8000 Patients. *Eur. Urol.* **2014**, *66*, 913–919. [CrossRef] [PubMed]
15. Afshar, N.; English, D.R.; Thursfield, V.; Mitchell, P.L.; Te Marvelde, L.; Farrugia, H.; Giles, G.G.; Milne, R.L. Differences in cancer survival by sex: A popula-tion-based study using cancer registry data. *Cancer Causes Control* **2018**, *29*, 1059–1069. [CrossRef] [PubMed]
16. Cook, M.B.; McGlynn, K.A.; Devesa, S.S.; Freedman, N.D.; Anderson, W.F. Sex Disparities in Cancer Mortality and Survival. *Cancer Epidemiol. Biomark. Prev.* **2011**, *20*, 1629–1637. [CrossRef] [PubMed]
17. Micheli, A.; Ciampichini, R.; Oberaigner, W.; Ciccolallo, L.; de Vries, E.; Izarzugaza, I.; Zambon, P.; Gatta, G.; De Angelis, R. The advantage of women in cancer survival: An analysis of EUROCARE-4 data. *Eur. J. Cancer* **2009**, *45*, 1017–1027. [CrossRef] [PubMed]
18. Lombard, A.P.; Mudryj, M. The emerging role of the androgen receptor in bladder cancer. *Endocr.-Relat. Cancer* **2015**, *22*, R265–R277. [CrossRef]
19. Cohn, J.A.; Vekhter, B.; Lyttle, C.; Steinberg, G.D.; Large, M.C. Sex disparities in diagnosis of bladder cancer after ini-tial presentation with hematuria: A nationwide claims-based investigation. *Cancer* **2014**, *120*, 555–561. [CrossRef]
20. Hollenbeck, B.K.; Ms, R.L.D.; Ye, Z.; Hollingsworth, J.M.; Skolarus, T.A.; Kim, S.P.; Montie, J.E.; Lee, C.T.; Wood, D.P.; Miller, D.C. Delays in diagnosis and bladder cancer mortality. *Cancer* **2010**, *116*, 5235–5242. [CrossRef]
21. Krimphove, M.J.; Szymaniak, J.; Marchese, M.; Tully, K.H.; D'Andrea, D.; Mossanen, M.; Lipsitz, S.R.; Kilbridge, K.; Kibel, A.S.; Kluth, L.A.; et al. Sex-specific Differences in the Quality of Treatment of Muscle-invasive Bladder Cancer Do Not Explain the Overall Survival Discrepancy. *Eur. Urol. Focus* **2021**, *7*, 124–131. [CrossRef] [PubMed]
22. Williams, S.B.; Huo, J.; Dafashy, T.J.; Ghaffary, C.K.; Baillargeon, J.G.; Morales, E.E.; Kim, S.P.; Kuo, Y.F.; Orihuela, E.; Tyler, D.S.; et al. Survival Differences among Bladder Cancer Patients Ac-cording to Gender: Critical Evaluation of Radical Cystectomy Use and Delay to Treatment. *Urol. Oncol.* **2017**, *35*, 602.e1. [CrossRef]
23. Jobczyk, M.; Pikala, M.; Różański, W.; Maniecka-Bryła, I. Years of life lost due to bladder cancer among the inhabitants of Poland in the years 2000 to 2014. *Central Eur. J. Urol.* **2017**, *70*, 338–343. [CrossRef]
24. Kimura, S.; Iwata, T.; Abufaraj, M.; Janisch, F.; D'Andrea, D.; Moschini, M.; Al-Rawashdeh, B.; Fajkovic, H.; Seebacher, V.; Egawa, S.; et al. Impact of Gender on Chemotherapeutic Response and Oncologic Out-comes in Patients Treated with Radical Cystectomy and Perioperative Chemotherapy for Bladder Cancer: A Sys-tematic Review and Meta-Analysis. *Clin. Genitourin. Cancer.* **2020**, *18*, 78–87. [CrossRef] [PubMed]
25. Choi, W.; Porten, S.; Kim, S.; Willis, D.; Plimack, E.R.; Hoffman-Censits, J.; Roth, B.; Cheng, T.; Tran, M.; Lee, I.-L; et al. Identification of Distinct Basal and Luminal Subtypes of Muscle-Invasive Bladder Cancer with Different Sensitivities to Frontline Chemotherapy. *Cancer Cell* **2014**, *25*, 152–165. [CrossRef]
26. Robertson, A.G.; Kim, J.; Al-Ahmadie, H.; Bellmunt, J.; Guo, G.; Cherniack, A.D.; Hinoue, T.; Laird, P.W.; Hoadley, K.A.; Akbani, R.; et al. Comprehensive Molecular Characterization of Mus-cle-Invasive Bladder Cancer. *Cell* **2017**, *171*, 540–556.e25. [CrossRef]
27. Seiler, R.; Ashab, H.A.D.; Erho, N.; van Rhijn, B.W.; Winters, B.; Douglas, J.; Van Kessel, K.E.; van de Putte, E.E.F.; Sommerlad, M.; Wang, N.Q.; et al. Impact of Molecular Subtypes in Muscle-invasive Bladder Cancer on Predicting Response and Survival after Neoadjuvant Chemotherapy. *Eur. Urol.* **2017**, *72*, 544–554. [CrossRef]
28. Volikova, A.I.; Marshall, B.J.; Yin, J.M.A.; Goodwin, R.; Chow, P.E.; Wise, M.J. Structural, biomechanical and hemodynamic assessment of the bladder wall in healthy sub-jects. *Res. Rep. Urol.* **2019**, *11*, 233–245.
29. James, A.C.; Lee, F.C.; Izard, J.; Harris, W.P.; Cheng, H.H.; Zhao, S.; Gore, J.; Lin, D.W.; Porter, M.P.; Yu, E.Y.; et al. Role of Maximal Endoscopic Resection Before Cystectomy for Invasive Urothelial Bladder Cancer. *Clin. Genitourin. Cancer* **2014**, *12*, 287–291. [CrossRef]

70. Pak, J.S.; Haas, C.R.; Anderson, C.B.; DeCastro, G.J.; Benson, M.C.; McKiernan, J.M. Survival and oncologic outcomes of complete transurethral resection of bladder tumor prior to neoadjuvant chemotherapy for muscle-invasive bladder cancer. *Urol. Oncol. Semin. Orig. Investig.* **2021**, *39*, 787.e9–787.e15. [CrossRef]
71. Haines, L.; Bamias, A.; Krege, S.; Lin, C.-C.; Hahn, N.; Ecke, T.H.; Moshier, E.; Sonpavde, G.; Godbold, J.; Oh, W.K.; et al. The Impact of Gender on Outcomes in Patients with Metastatic Urothelial Carcinoma. *Clin. Genitourin. Cancer* **2013**, *11*, 346–352. [CrossRef] [PubMed]
72. Porter, M.P.; Kerrigan, M.C.; Donato, B.M.; Ramsey, S.D. Patterns of use of systemic chemotherapy for Medicare beneficiaries with urothelial bladder cancer. *Urol Oncol.* **2011**, *29*, 252–258. [CrossRef] [PubMed]
73. D'Andrea, D.; Black, P.C.; Zargar, H.; Zargar-Shoshtari, K.; Zehetmayer, S.; Fairey, A.S.; Mertens, L.S.; Dinney, C.P.; Mir, M.C.; Krabbe, L.M.; et al. Impact of sex on response to neoadjuvant chem-otherapy in patients with bladder cancer. *Urol. Oncol. Semin. Orig. Investig.* **2020**, *38*, 639.e1–639.e9.
74. Venkat, S.; Khan, A.I.; Taylor, B.L.; Patel, N.A.; Al Hussein Al Awamlh, B.; Calderon, L.P.; Fainberg, J.; Shoag, J.; Scherr, D.S. Does neoadjuvant chemotherapy diminish the sex disparity in bladder cancer survival after radical cystectomy? *Urol. Oncol. Semin. Orig. Investig.* **2022**, *40*, 106.e21–106.e29. [CrossRef] [PubMed]
75. Barone, B.; Calogero, A.; Scafuri, L.; Ferro, M.; Lucarelli, G.; Di Zazzo, E.; Sicignano, E.; Falcone, A.; Romano, L.; De Luca, L.; et al. Immune Checkpoint Inhibitors as a Neoadju-vant/Adjuvant Treatment of Muscle-Invasive Bladder Cancer: A Systematic Review. *Cancers* **2022**, *14*, 2545. [CrossRef] [PubMed]
76. Iacovino, M.L.; Miceli, C.C.; De Felice, M.; Barone, B.; Pompella, L.; Chiancone, F.; Di Zazzo, E.; Tirino, G.; Della Corte, C.M.; Imbimbo, C.; et al. Novel Therapeutic Opportunities in Neoadjuvant Setting in Urothelial Cancers: A New Horizon Opened by Molecular Classification and Immune Checkpoint Inhibitors. *Int. J. Mol. Sci.* **2022**, *23*, 1133. [CrossRef] [PubMed]

Disclaimer/Publisher's Note: The statements, opinions and data contained in all publications are solely those of the individual author(s) and contributor(s) and not of MDPI and/or the editor(s). MDPI and/or the editor(s) disclaim responsibility for any injury to people or property resulting from any ideas, methods, instructions or products referred to in the content.

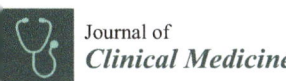

Article

Risk Factors Involved in the High Incidence of Bladder Cancer in an Industrialized Area in North-Eastern Spain: A Case–Control Study

José M. Caballero [1,2,*], José M. Gili [1], Juan C. Pereira [1], Alba Gomáriz [1], Carlos Castillo [1] and Montserrat Martín-Baranera [2,3]

1. Department of Urology, Hospital Universitari Mútua Terrassa, Plaza Dr. Robert 5, 08221 Terrassa, Spain
2. Department of Paediatrics, Obstetrics & Gynaecology and Preventive Medicine and Public Health, School of Medicine, Autonomous University of Barcelona, Edificio M Campus Universitario UAB, 08193 Barcelona, Spain
3. Department of Clinical Epidemiology, Consorci Sanitari Integral, Avinguda Josep Molins 29-41, 08906 Hospitalet de Llobregat, Spain
* Correspondence: jcaballero@mutuaterrassa.es

Abstract: Bladder cancer (BC) is the most common of the malignancies affecting the urinary tract. Smoking and exposure to occupational and environmental carcinogens are responsible for most cases. Vallès Occidental is a highly industrialized area in north-eastern Spain with one of the highest incidences of BC in men. We carried out a case–control study in order to identify the specific risk factors involved in this area. Three hundred and six participants were included (153 cases BC and 153 controls matched for age and sex): in each group, 89.5% ($n = 137$) were male and the mean age was 71 years (range 30–91; SD = 10.6). There were no differences between groups in family history, body mass index, or dietary habits. Independent risk factors for CV were smoking (OR 2.08; 95% CI 1.30–3.32; $p = 0.002$), the use of analgesics in nonsmokers (OR 10.00; 95% CI 1.28–78.12; $p = 0.028$), and profession (OR: 8.63; 95% CI 1.04–71.94; $p = 0.046$). The consumption of black and blond tobacco, the use of analgesics in nonsmokers, and occupational exposures are risk factors for the development of BC in this area, despite the reduction in smoking in the population and the extensive measures taken in the last few decades in major industries to prevent exposure to occupational carcinogens.

Keywords: bladder cancer; risk factors; occupational exposure; smoking; analgesics

1. Introduction

Bladder cancer (BC) is the most common of those affecting the urinary tract. Worldwide, BC is the seventh most common cancer diagnosed in men and the seventeenth in women. When only developed countries are considered, it ranks fourth and ninth in men and women, respectively. BC represents 4.4% of all new cancer diagnoses (excluding nonmelanoma skin cancer) in the United States and Europe [1].

The incidence of BC in Spain, adjusted for age to the Standard European Population, is 20.08 cases per 100,000 inhabitants (95% CI 13.9–26.3), one of the highest in Europe [2,3]. Vallès Occidental is a region of Catalonia located in the northeast of Spain with an extended industrial tradition, mainly textiles, in which a markedly elevated incidence of BC was detected in men in the 1990s [4]. This trend remains at present [5], with a crude rate of 62.6 (95% CI 55.0–70.1) in men and 6.8 (95% CI 4.4–9.3) in women, and an annual rate adjusted for the standard European population of 85.3 (95% CI 75.0–95.5) in men and 7.0 (95% CI 4.5–9.5) in women. In addition, although we do not have specific data on other types of cancer, the crude rate per 1000 inhabitants of active neoplasia in West Vallès Occidental in 2015 was significantly higher than that of the rest of Catalonia (29.17 vs. 21.85, respectively) [6].

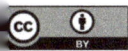

The main risk factor for the development of bladder cancer is smoking, accounting for 50% of the cases [7,8]. The occupational exposure to carcinogens is the second most relevant risk factor, the estimation being that up to 10% of bladder cancers have their origin in occupational exposure [9].

Given the high incidence of BC in Vallès Occidental, the current study aims to identify the independent risk factors that may favour the development of BC in this setting.

2. Materials and Methods

A case–control study was designed to assess BC risk factors. Cases were identified in the area of the Hospital Universitari Mútua Terrassa, which serves a population of more than 260,000 inhabitants; inclusion criteria were being aged 18 years or more, and having a histologically confirmed diagnosis of primary BC during the years 2018–2019. Controls were obtained from hospital-recruited individuals without BC, matched with cases for sex and age (± 2 years), during the same period. Both the cases and the controls had to be residents of the West Vallès Occidental health area. Cases with nonurothelial bladder tumors and recurrences were excluded from the study.

A sample size of at least 106 cases and 106 controls matched for age and sex was estimated, accepting an alpha risk of 0.05 and a beta risk of 0.2 in a bilateral contrast, to detect a minimum odds ratio of 2.5. It was assumed that the proportion of exposure to any of the studied factors in the control group would be 0.2 [10].

A survey was developed to obtain information through a direct interview, always conducted by the same urologist, who inquired about the patient's demographic and medical data, as well as about the risk factors under study. Possible risk factors included medical family history of BC; area of habitual residence; consumption of toxic substances, including black and blond tobacco (number of cigarettes per day and years of consumption) and alcohol intake (grams of alcohol per day and years of consumption); characteristics of diet in relation to the consumption of caffeinated or decaffeinated coffee (number of cups of coffee and years of consumption), intake of water from the public network or bottled (litters of water per day) and habitual consumption of animal fats; and analgesic intake. Subjects were asked if they used an analgesic at least once a week for a month or more before the date of inclusion in the study (date of diagnosis of BC in the cases). Those who responded positively were asked about the number of weekly analgesic tablets and the condition for which the drug was prescribed.

Finally, both current and past occupational exposures and years of exposure to each of them were recorded. After a descriptive analysis of every occupational exposure, both in cases and controls, the assessment of professions as a BC risk factor was based on a meta-analysis of 263 articles [11], in which 61 occupations were classified following the codes of the International Standard Classification of Occupations (ISCO-58) [12]; the corresponding odds ratio (OR) for BC for every employment was then estimated: 42 occupations showed an increased incidence of BC, while 6 had a lower incidence. In the present study, and for analysis purposes, to summarize the different occupations collected along the participants' working history, we assigned to every case and control the maximum risk of occupational exposure, expressed as the corresponding OR estimated in the above-mentioned meta-analysis [11].

This study was approved by the Ethics and Research Committee of the Hospital Universitari Mútua de Terrassa and conformed to the principles of the Declaration of Helsinki. All participants signed informed consent.

The statistical analysis of the data was carried out using the IBM SPSS version 26 program, including measures of central tendency and dispersion for the quantitative variables, and the frequencies with the corresponding percentages for the qualitative variables. For all the variables (risk factors) collected, the OR was initially obtained by means of a conditional logistic regression model, to account for matching, in which the dependent variable was a case or a control. The factors that showed statistical significance in the bivariate analysis were afterwards included in a multivariate conditional logistic regression model to obtain the corresponding adjusted OR and their 95% confidence intervals. In this model, the possible interaction between tobacco, coffee, and analgesic consumption was explored.

3. Results

A total of 306 participants were included in the study: 153 cases and 153 controls matched for age and sex. In each group, 89.5% ($n = 137$) of the participants were male. The mean age was 71.98 years (range 30–91; SD = 10.64) for the cases and 71.91 years (range 30–91; SD = 10.62) for the controls. The age distribution was identical in both groups, with 76.5% ($n = 117$) older than 65 years.

3.1. Family Background

There were no significant differences between cases and controls in terms of the presence of family history (68.8% vs. 31.3%, $p = 0.123$) (Table 1) nor globally (OR = 2.20; 95% CI 0.76–6.33) (Table 2).

Table 1. Bivariate assessment of risk factors involved in bladder cancer in West Vallès Occidental.

	Variable	Cases	Controls	*p*-Value [1]
Family background of bladder cancer	n (%)	11 (68.8)	5 (31.3)	0.123
Obesity (BMI > 30)	n (%)	47 (30,7)	42 (27.5)	0.615
Blond tobacco	n (%) Number cigarettes/day. mean (SD) Years, mean (SD)	81 (52.94) 21.64 (12.10) 35.95 (13.69)	53 (34.64) 15.64 (8.77) 29.74 (15.73)	**0.001** **0.002** **0.017**
Black tobacco	n (%) Number cigarettes/day. mean (SD) Years, mean(SD)	68 (44.44) 21.99 (14.81) 36.13 (16.24)	38 (24.84) 18.37 (11.71) 32.13 (14.67)	**<0.0001** 0.198 0.211
Caffeinated coffee	n (%) Number cups of coffee/day. mean (SD) Years, mean (SD)	122 (79.74) 2.04 (1.58) 47.84 (20.78)	111 (72.55) 2.05 (1.33) 45.92 (11.82)	0.141 0.946 0.392
Decaffeinated coffee	n (%) Number cups of coffee/day mean (SD) Years, mean (SD)	24 (15.69) 2.33 (1.71) 32.67 (18.67)	24 (15.69) 1.54 (0.93) 45.79 (12.86)	1.000 0.052 **0.007**
Alcohol consumption	n (%) Grams of alcohol/day. mean (SD) Years. Mean (SD)	101 (66.01) 38.22 (26.24) 47.90 (10.87)	98 (64.05) 31.33 (21.44) 47.61 (9.56)	0.720 **0.044** 0.843
Tap water	n (%) Liters/day, mean (SD)	53 (34.64) 1.82 (2.07)	47 (30.72) 1.28 (0.51)	0.465 0.086
Bottled water	n (%) Liters/day, mean (SD)	101 (66.01) 2.02 (3.09)	107 (69.93) 1.27 (0.53)	0.463 **0.013**
Animal fats	n (%) Quantity, mean (SD)	141 (92.16) 2.96 (1.64)	146 (95.42) 3.09 (1.70)	0.237 0.52
Analgesics treatments	n (%) Tablets/week, mean (SD)	58 (37.91) 6.83 (2.33)	28 (18.30) 6.36 (1.64)	**<0.0001** 0.34

n = number of individuals; SD: standard deviation. [1] Student *t* test for parametric variables and Mann–Whitney U for nonparametric variables, significance level <0.05. **In bold**, significant *p*-values.

Table 2. Odds ratio and 95% CI for the risk factors collected.

Variable	Conditional Logistic Regression	
	OR (95% CI)	p
Age	1.16 (0.83–1.63)	0.393
Family background of bladder cancer	2.20 (0.76–6.33)	0.144
Body mass index (BMI)	1.03 (0.98–1.09)	0.217
Obesity (BMI > 30)	1.17 (0.71–1.92)	0.529
Blond tobacco	**2.08 (1.30–3.32)**	**0.002**
Black tobacco	**2.67 (1.55–4.58)**	**<0.0001**
Caffeinated coffee	1.61 (0.89–2.90)	0.112
Decaffeinated coffee	1.00 (0.51–1.96)	1.000
Alcohol consumption	1.11 (0.66–1.87)	0.691
Tap water	1.18 (0.74–1.88)	0.480
Bottled water	0.85 (0.53–1.34)	0.480
Animal fats	1.83 (0.68–4.96)	0.232
Analgesics treatments	**2.67 (1.55–4.58)**	**<0.0001**

OR = odds ratio; 95% CI = 95% confidence interval for OR. **In bold**, significant *p*-values OR (significance level < 0.05).

3.2. Body Mass Index

No differences in body mass index (BMI) were observed between either group. Mean BMI was 28.62 ± 4.24 in cases and 28.04 ± 3.93 in controls ($p = 0.21$). The percentage of patients with obesity (BMI > 30) was similar between groups (30.7% in cases; 27.5% in controls; $p = 0.615$) (Table 1).

3.3. Smoking

On the one hand, blond tobacco was a risk factor for developing BC (OR 2.08; 95% CI 1.30–3.32; $p = 0.002$). The proportion of blond tobacco smokers was statistically different between cases and controls (52.94%, $n = 81$ vs. 34.64%, $n = 53$; $p = 0.001$). The differences remained statistically significant between groups when comparing the number of cigarettes per day ($p = 0.002$) and the years they have been smoking ($p = 0.017$). On the other hand, black tobacco was also a risk factor for developing BC (OR 2.67; 95% CI 1.55–4.58; $p < 0.0001$) (Tables 1 and 2). Significant differences were found in the proportion of black tobacco smoking between cases and controls (44.44% ($n = 68$) vs. 24.84% ($n = 38$), $p < 0.0001$) However, no significant differences were observed in the number of daily cigarettes and the years of consumption of black tobacco in smokers of both groups.

3.4. Diet

The proportion of subjects consuming caffeinated or decaffeinated coffee, alcohol, tap or bottled water, and animal fats did not statistically differ between cases and controls Controls had been consuming decaffeinated coffee for more years than cases ($p = 0.007$) Among the subjects who consumed alcohol, the patients with BC had a higher daily alcohol intake than those in the control group ($p = 0.044$), without any differences in the years of consumption. Overall, no variables related to diet seemed to behave as risk factors for developing BC (Tables 1 and 2).

3.5. Analgesics Treatments

Eighty-six subjects were taking analgesics (seven tablets weekly in 73 subjects). There was a statistically significant difference in the consumption of analgesics between the cases (37.91%, n = 58) and the controls (18.30%, n = 28) (p < 0.0001) (Table 1). Analgesic consumption was a risk factor for developing BC (OR 2.67; 95% CI 1.55–4.58) (Table 2). None of the subjects had been prescribed pain-relieving drugs for BC.

To explore the possible interaction between tobacco, coffee consumption, and analgesics, first-order interaction terms were included in a conditional logistic regression model. The interaction between tobacco and coffee was not significant (neither for the global coffee variable, nor for the caffeinated coffee variable); in contrast, a significant interaction between tobacco and analgesics was pointed out (p = 0.012). Therefore, conditional odds ratios for coffee and analgesic consumption were estimated after stratifying by smoking (Table 3). In that way, analgesics showed a statistically significant association with bladder cancer in nonsmokers (OR 10.00; 95% CI 1.28–78.12; p = 0.028) but not in smokers (OR= 1.080; 95% CI 0.83–3.90; p = 0.136).

Table 3. Estimated odds ratios for coffee and analgesics consumption as risk factors for bladder cancer, stratified by smoking status.

Variable	Cases (n = 152) n (No/Yes)	Controls (n = 152) n (No/Yes)	Nonsmoker		Smoker	
			OR (95% CI)	p-Value [1]	OR (95% CI)	p-Value [1]
Coffee consumption	17/136	24/129	1.00 (0.14–7.10)	1.000	0.43 (0.11–1.66)	0.220
Caffeinated coffee consumption	31/122	42/111	1.50 (0.25–8.98)	0.657	0.82 (0.34–1.97)	0.655
Analgesics treatment	95/58	125/28	**10.00 (1.28–78.12)**	**0.028**	1.80 (0.83–3.90)	0.136

Odds ratios (OR) and 95% confidence intervals (95% CI) were estimated by means of conditional logistic regression. In bold, p-values and significant OR ([1] significance level < 0.05).

3.6. Occupational Exposure

When recording work history both in cases and controls, many different occupations were listed, leading to very small numbers in most of the professions (Table 4). Due to this high variability of working settings, the role of occupational exposure in relation to bladder cancer was assessed by using the previously defined variable, which assigned to each subject the estimated OR corresponding to the profession with the maximum estimated occupational risk for BC. Therefore, the occupational level of estimated risk of BC ranged in the study sample from 0.69 to 1.58, with percentiles 25, 50, and 75 being 1.10, 1.11, and 1.17, respectively. There was a statistically significant association between bladder cancer (being case or control) and the occupational level of risk for BC (OR = 6.72; 95% CI 1.06–42.7; p = 0.043). More than 75% of the cases and controls were retired at the time of inclusion in the study (76.47% in cases and 78.43 in controls, p = 0.682).

Table 4. Comparison between cases and controls of the different types of occupation and the years spent.

Occupational		Cases	Controls	p-Value [1]
Homemaker	n (%)	7	1	**0.032**
	Mean years (SD)	49.14 (13.09)	60	0.467
Textile	n (%)	30	21	0.167
	Mean years (SD)	24.70 (16.79)	27.95 (18.14)	0.513
Mechanic	n (%)	17	9	0.102
	Mean years (SD)	26.65 (19.93)	20.78 (14.90)	0.447
Truck driver	n (%)	9	12	0.652
	Mean years (SD)	20.67 (13.53)	28.92 (14.38)	0.198
Painter	n (%)	9	5	0.275
	Mean years (SD)	26.89 (19.20)	20.40 (13.76)	0.520

Table 4. Cont.

Occupational		Cases	Controls	p-Value [1]
Rubber-plastic	n (%)	3	1	0.623
	Mean years (SD)	9.67 (8.39)	39.00	0.094
Asbestos	n (%)	2	0	0.498
	Mean years (SD)	9.00 (9.90)	-	-
Printing	n (%)	5	3	0.723
	Mean years (SD)	36.00 (20.16)	40.00 (12.77)	0.772
Agriculture	n (%)	17	8	0.093
	Mean years (SD)	13.29 (10.60)	8.75 (2.05)	0.247
Laundry	n (%)	1	-	-
	Mean years (SD)	6.00	-	-
Building	n (%)	30	28	0.884
	Mean years (SD)	31.17 (17.88)	24.36 (17.87)	0.153
Welder	n (%)	2	2	1.00
	Mean years (SD)	46.00 (5.66)	30.00 (21.21)	0.411
Hairdressing	n (%)	1	3	0.315
	Mean years (SD))	8.00	35.67 (23.12)	0.409
Dyes	n (%)	2	0	0.498
	Mean years (SD)	3.50 (0.70)		-
Metallurgy	n (%)	17	24	0.314
	Mean years (SD)	21.82 (12.04)	26.67 (19.76)	0.375
Chemistry	n (%)	7	6	0.777
	Mean years (SD)	25.71 (13.99)	34.67 (16.70)	0.315
Mining	n (%)	1	0	1.00
	Mean years (SD)	2.00		
Fire-fighter	n (%)	0	1	1.00
	Mean years (SD)		35.00	-
Electricity	n (%)	5	53	1.00
	Mean years (SD))	33.00 (17.19)	1.80 (14.38)	0.908
Feeding	n (%)	4	8	0.378
	Mean years (SD)	12.75 (15.15)	22.62 (15.24)	0.314
Sales	n (%)	20	22	0.740
	Mean years (SD))	29.35 (15.94)	30.14 (16.27)	0.875
Waiter	n (%)	7	7	1.00
	Mean years (SD)	19.57 (15.10)	16.00 (15.71)	0.672
Health area	n (%)	5	5	1.00
	Mean years (SD)	35.60 (11.54)	20 (11.25)	0.062
Office	n (%)	18	21	0.732
	Mean years (SD)	35.61 (14.62)	38.24 (13.84)	0.568
Teaching	n (%)	1	10	**0.010**
	Mean years (SD)	4.00	36.40 (5.08)	**<0.0001**
Others	n (%)	29	32	0.775
	Mean years (SD)	29.03 (14.40)	32.66 (15.67)	0.353

n = number of individuals; [1] **In bold**, p-value and significant OR (significance level <0.05).

3.7. Multivariable Model

Finally, factors that have shown a statistically significant association with being a case of BC in the bivariate analysis were considered for inclusion in a multivariable conditional logistic regression model (Table 5). Adjusted by tobacco consumption and intake of analgesics, the occupational level of exposure was an independent risk factor for the development of BC (OR: 8.63, 95% CI 1.04–71.94, $p = 0.046$).

Table 5. Independent predictive factors of bladder cancer. Conditional logistic regression model.

	B	p-Value [1]	OR	95.0% CI for OR	
				Lower	Upper
Occupational risk	2.156	**0.046**	8.634	1.036	71.941
Blond tobacco	1.272	**<0.0001**	3.567	1.917	6.639
Dark tobacco	1.448	**<0.0001**	4.255	2.178	8.311
Analgesics	0.912	**0.004**	2.490	1.336	4.643

[1] In **bold**, p-values and significant OR (significance level <0.05).

4. Discussion

The incidence of BC in Vallès Occidental remains one of the highest in men and one of the lowest in women, at a European and global level, despite the decline in tobacco consumption and industrial activity over the years [6]. Compared to data published during the period 1992–1994, both the crude annual incidence and age-adjusted incidence have increased in both sexes, although the increase in men is notably higher [5,13]. The high incidence of BC in men, some 25 years later, could be related to a high prevalence in this area of well-known risk factors such as smoking, residence in industrialized areas, and occupational exposure to certain carcinogenic products [13,14]. The analysis of possible environmental factors involved in this area showed that although the annual average concentrations of possible air and water pollutants were within the regulatory limit values, the maximum levels detected were usually higher than what was established [6]. In this case–control study, we try to identify other risk factors specifically related to BC in our health area.

The genetic involvement in bladder cancer is becoming increasingly well known. The risk of BC is twice as high in first-degree relatives of patients with BC, in relation to certain inherited genetic factors [7,15]. However, because of a lack of statistical power, the current results did not find significant differences between cases and controls in the presence of family history.

Smoking is also an important risk factor for BC in our area, both for dark tobacco and blond tobacco. Interestingly, both the number of daily cigarettes consumed and the years of smoking are significantly higher in the cases than in the controls for light tobacco, but not for dark tobacco. Although dark tobacco had traditionally been attributed a much higher risk than blond tobacco, the largest study to evaluate the effects of dark tobacco versus the use of blond tobacco on BC in Spain showed that the risk was only 40% higher for dark tobacco smokers compared to blond tobacco smokers, and this difference was not statistically significant [16]. In addition, smoking continues to be an important risk factor in our environment despite a significant decreased prevalence over time [6]. In Catalonia, in 1994, the prevalence of smokers in the population over 15 years of age was 42.3% in men and 20.7% in women. In 2018, the prevalence in men decreased to 30.9, although it remained high in the 35–44 age group (40.3%). In women, however, the 2018 prevalence of smoking was unchanged (20.5%), the highest figures being found between 25–34 years (31.6%). Previous studies showed that only 15.1% of the BC cases diagnosed during 1993–1995 in the Vallès Occidental had never smoked [13,17].

Various dietary factors have been investigated in numerous studies as likely risk factors for developing BC, with conflicting results. Although a higher fluid intake has been suggested to reduce the incidence of BC by diluting carcinogenic substances and promoting more frequent urination, thus limiting their effect on urothelial cells, studies focused on this hypothesis have not been able to validate it [18,19]. The chlorination of water, with the consequent level of trihalomethanes, has been considered an important carcinogenic risk of BC [20], and some studies have cited a higher BC risk in consumers of tap water due to the presence of trihalomethanes [21], or even as a risk factor independently of the chlorination [22]. Traditionally, coffee intake had been associated with a slight increase in the incidence of BC in smokers [22]. A recent meta-analysis of 10 cohorts and some case–control studies found no evidence of an association between BC and coffee intake [23], nor has alcohol has been shown to be a risk factor for BC [24]. Finally, some studies have observed a relationship between the consumption of processed meat and animal proteins, and an increased risk of BC [25,26]. We have not found differences between cases and controls in any risk factor related to diet (consumption of coffee, alcohol, bottled or tap water, and animal fats). The fact that the subjects in the control group had been consuming decaffeinated coffee for more years could suggest a doubtful protective effect against BC.

Overweight and obesity have been described as risk factors in BC [27]. BMI has been associated with a linear rise in BC, with risk increasing by 4.2% for each increase of 5 mg/m^2. However, this relationship may be biased by the fact that high BMIs are related to bad habits, such as little physical activity and inadequate diet [28]. In our study, we found no relationship between BC and BMI.

The association between the use of different types of analgesics and BC risk is controversial. On the one hand, there was strong experimental and epidemiological evidence that nonsteroidal anti-inflammatory drugs (NSAIDs) and cyclooxygenase 2 (COX-2) inhibitors might have a potential as cancer chemopreventive agents [29]. For example, ibuprofen, naproxen, indomethacin, piroxicam, and celecoxib inhibit BC development in a variety of human and animal models [29,30]. However, other studies describe an increased risk of BC associated with the use of phenacetin-containing analgesics, particularly with longer use There are doubts about the association of paracetamol with BC, even though it is a metabolite of phenacetin [31,32]. Nor was regular use of any NSAID, including aspirin, associated with a statistically significant lower BC risk [31]. In a meta-analysis that included 17 articles on BC risk and analgesic use (8 cohort studies and 9 case–control studies), with a total of 10,618 cases of bladder cancer, there was no significant association between paracetamol use, aspirin, or other types of NSAIDs and BC risk [33]. However, NSAID use has been significantly associated with a 43% reduction in BC risk among nonsmokers but not among active smokers [15]. COX-2 expression is associated with increased tumor development. In smokers, both the expression and the activity of COX-2 are increased in urothelial tissues, but the anticancer effects of NSAIDs against COX-2 seem to be counteracted by the carcinogenic effect of smoking [34]. Our study did not show any protective effect of analgesics. In addition, the use of analgesics was related to BC in nonsmokers, thus being a risk factor independent of tobacco.

Occupational exposure to carcinogens such as aromatic amines (benzidine, 4-aminobiphenyl, 2-naphthylamine, 4-chloro-o-toluidine), polycyclic aromatic hydrocarbons, and chlorinated hydrocarbons, is considered the second most important risk factor for BC after smoking [9,11,15]. Approximately 20–25% of all BC are related to such exposure, mainly in industrial areas where paint, dyes, rubber, textiles, leather, metals, and petroleum products are processed, with a latency period of several decades [35]. Although in recent years the extent and pattern of occupational exposure have drastically changed due to an improved awareness of occupational safety measures [9], some occupations, such as those in the chemical sector, are still considered as risk factors; rubber, textile, printing, and other industries are probably linked to exposure to carcinogenic agents. The relationship of BC with hair dye, or even with the hairdressing professional who handles such products, is still controversial [9].

In our environment, our data pointed to profession as a risk factor for developing BC, independently of tobacco and analgesics consumption. A meta-analysis of 263 publications [11] concluded that although there is evidence of a decrease in the incidence and occupational mortality of BC, certain occupations are still associated with a high incidence or greater risk of mortality from BC: there is an increase in the incidence of BC in 42 of 61 occupations analyzed and of BC-specific mortality in 16 of 40, although not all studies had explored specific mortality. The highest combined incidence risks are seen in tobacco workers (RR 1.72, 95% CI 1.37–2.15) and dye workers (RR 13.4, 95% CI 1.5–48.2). However, the highest RR reported in any study was for factory workers overall (RR 16.6; 95% CI, 2.1–131.3). In terms of grouped disease-specific mortality, it is higher for metal workers (RR, 10.2; 95% CI, 6.89–15.09) and gardeners (RR, 5.5; 95% CI, 0.84–35.89) with the highest disease-specific mortality reported in any study for chemical workers (RR, 27.1; 95% CI, 11.7–53.4) [11]. These high BC incidences and mortality persist despite improvements in workplace safety measures, and efforts to reduce the impact of BC on workers should be directed at the highest-risk occupations.

The textile industry constituted the economic base of the Vallès Occidental region from the mid-19th century to the 1970s. This fact justified the performance of BC incidence and population-based case–control studies whose objectives were to assess occupational risk factors for BC in this area [5,13,17]. These studies demonstrated that tobacco consumption was strongly associated with BC [13]. However, when analyzing BC risk associated with exposure in the textile industry as part of a large case–control study carried out in five areas of Spain (Asturias, Alicante, Barcelona, Tenerife and Vallès/Bages), working in the textile industry was not associated with a higher BC risk. However, specific occupations within the textile industry (for example, weavers) and specific locations (winding, warping and gluing, and weaving room), as well as having contact with specific materials (synthetics and cotton), showed an increased BC risk [14].

A limitation of this case–control study is the small sample size, which does not allow us to make comparisons between men and women in terms of tobacco consumption, use of analgesics, and professions. It would also have been interesting to have information on the type of analgesics being consumed, to assess the differences between steroidal drugs and NSAIDs.

5. Conclusions

We conclude that consumption of black and blond tobacco, the use of analgesics in nonsmoking patients, and profession are independent risk factors for the development of BC in our environment. The decline in smoking in the population, especially in men, and the improvements in job security have not been sufficient to reduce this high incidence of BC.

Author Contributions: J.M.C. and M.M.-B. contributed to the study conception and design. J.M.C. contributed to data collection. J.M.C. and M.M.-B. were responsible for data analysis and data interpretation. J.M.C. and M.M.-B. were responsible for manuscript writing. J.M.G., J.C.P., A.G. and C.C. Authors have read and corrected the final version of the manuscript. All authors have read and agreed to the published version of the manuscript.

Funding: This research received no external funding.

Institutional Review Board Statement: The study was conducted according to the guidelines of the Declaration of Helsinki, and approved by the Ethics and Research Committee of the Hospital Universitari Mútua de Terrassa (date of approval 18 July 2018).

Informed Consent Statement: Informed consent was obtained from all subjects involved in the study.

Data Availability Statement: Data sharing is not applicable to this article as no datasets were generated or analyzed during the current study.

Acknowledgments: This research has been carried out within the framework of the doctoral program of Methodology of Biomedical Research and Public Health at the Department of Pediatrics, Obstetrics & Gynecology and Preventative Medicine at the Autonomous University of Barcelona.

Conflicts of Interest: The authors declare no conflict of interest.

References

1. Babjuk, M.; Oosterlinck, W.; Sylvester, R.; Kaasinen, E.; Böhle, A.; Palou-Redorta, J.; Rouprêt, M.; European Association of Urology (EAU). EAU guidelines on non-muscle-invasive urothelial carcinoma of the bladder, the 2011 update. *Eur. Urol.* **2011**, *59*, 997–1008. [CrossRef] [PubMed]
2. Miñana, B.; Cózar, J.M.; Palou, J.; Urzaiz, M.U.; Medina-Lopez, R.A.; Ríos, J.S.; de la Rosa-Kehrmann, F.; Chantada-Abal, V.; Lozano, F.; Ribal, M.J.; et al. Bladder cancer in Spain 2011: Population based study. *J. Urol.* **2014**, *191*, 323–328. [CrossRef] [PubMed]
3. Antoni, S.; Ferlay, J.; Soerjomataram, I.; Znaor, A.; Jemal, A.; Bray, F. Bladder Cancer Incidence and Mortality: A Global Overview and Recent Trends. *Eur. Urol.* **2017**, *71*, 96–108. [CrossRef] [PubMed]
4. Urrutia, G.; Serra, C.; Bonfill, X.; Bastús, R.; Grupo Trabajo para el Estudio del Cáncer de Vejiga Urinaria en la Comarca del Vallès Occidental. Incidencia del cáncer de vejiga urinaria en un área industrializada de España [Incidence of urinary bladder cancer in an industrialized area of Spain]. *Gac. Sanit.* **2002**, *16*, 291–297. [CrossRef] [PubMed]
5. Caballero, J.M.; Pérez-Márquez, M.; Gili, J.M.; Pereira, J.C.; Gomáriz, A.; Castillo, C.; Martin-Baranera, M. Environmental Factors Involved in the High Incidence of Bladder Cancer in an Industrialized Area in North-Eastern Spain. *J. Environ. Public Health* **2022**, *2022*, 1051046. [CrossRef]
6. Departament de Salut, Generalitat de Catalunya. *Servei Català de la Salut. Pla Estratègic Sanitari del Vallès Occidental 2017–2020. Part B. Anàlisi de Situación [Vallès Occidental Health Strategic Plan 2017–2020. Part B. Situation Analysis]*; Barcelona Institute for Global Health: Barcelona, Spain, 2018.
7. Burger, M.; Catto, J.W.; Dalbagni, G.; Grossman, H.B.; Herr, H.; Karakiewicz, P.; Kassouf, W.; Kiemeney, L.A.; La Vecchia, C.; Shariat, S.; et al. Epidemiology and risk factors of urothelial bladder cancer. *Eur. Urol.* **2013**, *63*, 234–241. [CrossRef]
8. Freedman, N.D.; Silverman, D.T.; Hollenbeck, A.R.; Schatzkin, A.; Abnet, C.C. Association between smoking and risk of bladder cancer among men and women. *JAMA.* **2011**, *17*, 737–745. [CrossRef]
9. Anttila, S.; Boffetta, P. *Occupational Cancers*, 2nd ed.; Springer Nature: Cham, Switzerland, 2020. [CrossRef]
10. Farzaneh, F.; Mehrparvar, A.H.; Lotfi, M.H. Occupations and the Risk of Bladder Cancer in Yazd Province: A Case-Control Study. *Int. J. Occup. Environ. Med.* **2017**, *8*, 191–198. [CrossRef]
11. Cumberbatch, M.G.; Cox, A.; Teare, D.; Catto, J.W. Contemporary Occupational Carcinogen Exposure and Bladder Cancer: A Systematic Review and Meta-analysis. *JAMA. Oncol.* **2015**, *1*, 1282–1290. [CrossRef]
12. Pukkala, E.; Martinsen, J.I.; Lynge, E.; Gunnarsdottir, H.K.; Sparén, P.; Tryggvadottir, L.; Weiderpass, E.; Kjaerheim, K. Occupation and cancer-follow-up of 15 million people in five Nordic countries. *Acta Oncol.* **2009**, *48*, 646–790. [CrossRef]
13. Serra, C. Ocupació i Càncer de Bufeta Urinària al Vallès Occidental. [Occupation and Bladder Cancer in the Vallès Occidental]. Ph.D. Thesis, Autonomous University of Barcelona, Barcelona, Spain, 2002. Available online: http://hdl.handle.net/10803/4587 (accessed on 3 June 2020). (In Catalan)
14. Serra, C.; Kogevinas, M.; Silverman, D.T.; Turuguet, D.; Tardon, A.; Garcia-Closas, R.; Carrato, A.; Castaño-Vinyals, G.; Fernandez, F.; Stewart, P.; et al. Work in the textile industry in Spain and bladder cancer. *Occup. Environ. Med.* **2008**, *65*, 552–559. [CrossRef]
15. Cumberbatch, M.G.K.; Jubber, I.; Black, P.C.; Esperto, F.; Figueroa, J.D.; Kamat, A.M.; Kiemeney, L.; Lotan, Y.; Pang, K.; Silverman, D.T.; et al. Epidemiology of Bladder Cancer: A Systematic Review and Contemporary Update of Risk Factors in 2018. *Eur. Urol.* **2018**, *74*, 784–795. [CrossRef]
16. Samanic, C.; Kogevinas, M.; Dosemeci, M.; Malats, N.; Real, F.X.; Garcia-Closas, M.; Serra, C.; Carrato, A.; García-Closas, R.; Sala, M.; et al. Smoking and bladder cancer in Spain: Effects of tobacco type, timing, environmental tobacco smoke, and gender. *Cancer Epidemiol. Biomark. Prev.* **2006**, *15*, 1348–1354. [CrossRef]
17. Serra, C.; Bonfill, X.; Sunyer, J.; Urrutia, G.; Turuguet, D.; Bastús, R.; Roqué, M.; Mannetje, A.; Kogevinas, M.; Working Group on the Study of Bladder Cancer in the County of Vallès Occidental. Bladder cancer in the textile industry. *Scand. J. Work Environ. Health* **2000**, *26*, 476–481. [CrossRef]
18. Zhou, J.; Kelsey, K.T.; Giovannucci, E.; Michaud, D.S. Fluid intake and risk of bladder cancer in the Nurses' Health Studies. *Int. J. Cancer* **2014**, *135*, 1229–1237. [CrossRef]
19. Liu, Q.; Liao, B.; Tian, Y.; Chen, Y.; Luo, D.; Lin, Y.; Li, H.; Wang, K.J. Total fluid consumption and risk of bladder cancer: A meta-analysis with updated data. *Oncotarget* **2017**, *8*, 55467–55477. [CrossRef]
20. Michaud, D.S.; Kogevinas, M.; Cantor, K.P.; Villanueva, C.M.; Garcia-Closas, M.; Rothman, N.; Malats, N.; Real, F.X.; Serra, C.; Garcia-Closas, R.; et al. Total fluid and water consumption and the joint effect of exposure to disinfection by-products on risk of bladder cancer. *Environ. Health Perspect.* **2007**, *115*, 1569–1572. [CrossRef]
21. Villanueva, C.M.; Cantor, K.P.; Cordier, S.; Jaakkola, J.J.; King, W.D.; Lynch, C.F.; Porru, S.; Kogevinas, M. Disinfection byproducts and bladder cancer: A pooled analysis. *Epidemiology* **2004**, *15*, 357–367. [CrossRef]
22. Villanueva, C.M.; Cantor, K.P.; Grimalt, J.O.; Malats, N.; Silverman, D.; Tardon, A.; Garcia-Closas, R.; Serra, C.; Carrato, A.; Castaño-Vinyals, G.; et al. Bladder cancer and exposure to water disinfection by-products through ingestion, bathing, showering, and swimming in pools. *Am. J. Epidemiol.* **2007**, *165*, 148–156. [CrossRef]
23. Loomis, D.; Guyton, K.Z.; Grosse, Y.; Lauby-Secretan, B.; El Ghissassi, F.; Bouvard, V.; Benbrahim-Tallaa, L.; Guha, N.; Mattock, H.; Straif, K.; et al. Carcinogenicity of drinking coffee, mate, and very hot beverages. *Lancet Oncol.* **2016**, *17*, 877–878. [CrossRef]

4. Botteri, E.; Ferrari, P.; Roswall, N.; Tjønneland, A.; Hjartåker, A.; Huerta, J.M.; Fortner, R.T.; Trichopoulou, A.; Karakatsani, A.; La Vecchia, C.; et al. Alcohol consumption and risk of urothelial cell bladder cancer in the European prospective investigation into cancer and nutrition cohort. *Int. J. Cancer* **2017**, *141*, 1963–1970. [CrossRef] [PubMed]
5. Catsburg, C.E.; Gago-Dominguez, M.; Yuan, J.M.; Castelao, J.E.; Cortessis, V.K.; Pike, M.C.; Stern, M.C. Dietary sources of N-nitroso compounds and bladder cancer risk: Findings from the Los Angeles bladder cancer study. *Int. J. Cancer* **2014**, *134*, 125–135. [CrossRef] [PubMed]
6. Allen, N.E.; Appleby, P.N.; Key, T.J.; Bueno-de-Mesquita, H.B.; Ros, M.M.; Kiemeney, L.A.; Tjønneland, A.; Roswall, N.; Overvad, K.; Weikert, S.; et al. Macronutrient intake and risk of urothelial cell carcinoma in the European prospective investigation into cancer and nutrition. *Int. J. Cancer* **2013**, *132*, 635–644. [CrossRef] [PubMed]
7. Sun, J.W.; Zhao, L.G.; Yang, Y.; Ma, X.; Wang, Y.Y.; Xiang, Y.B. Obesity and risk of bladder cancer: A dose-response meta-analysis of 15 cohort studies. *PLoS ONE* **2015**, *10*, e0119313. [CrossRef] [PubMed]
8. Reulen, R.C.; de Vogel, S.; Zhong, W.; Zhong, Z.; Xie, L.P.; Hu, Z.; Deng, Y.; Yang, K.; Liang, Y.; Zeng, X.; et al. Physical activity and risk of prostate and bladder cancer in China: The South and East China case-control study on prostate and bladder cancer. *PLoS ONE* **2017**, *12*, e0178613. [CrossRef]
9. La Rochelle, J.; Kamat, A.; Grossman, H.B.; Pantuck, A. Chemoprevention of bladder cancer. *BJU. Int.* **2008**, *102*, 1274–1278. [CrossRef]
10. Liu, X.; Wu, Y.; Zhou, Z.; Huang, M.; Deng, W.; Wang, Y.; Zhou, X.; Chen, L.; Li, Y.; Zeng, T.; et al. Celecoxib inhibits the epithelial-to-mesenchymal transition in bladder cancer via the miRNA-145/TGFBR2/Smad3 axis. *Int. J. Mol. Med.* **2019**, *44*, 683–693. [CrossRef]
11. Fortuny, J.; Kogevinas, M.; Zens, M.S.; Schned, A.; Andrew, A.S.; Heaney, J.; Kelsey, K.T.; Karagas, M.R. Analgesic and anti-inflammatory drug use and risk of bladder cancer: A population based case control study. *BMC Urol.* **2007**, *7*, 13. [CrossRef]
12. Pommer, W.; Bronder, E.; Klimpel, A.; Helmert, U.; Greiser, E.; Molzahn, M. Urothelial cancer at different tumour sites: Role of smoking and habitual intake of analgesics and laxatives. Results of the Berlin Urothelial Cancer Study. *Nephrol. Dial. Transplant.* **1999**, *14*, 2892–2897. [CrossRef]
13. Zhang, H.; Jiang, D.; Li, X. Use of nonsteroidal anti-inflammatory drugs and bladder cancer risk: A meta-analysis of epidemiologic studies. *PLoS ONE* **2013**, *8*, e70008. [CrossRef]
14. Badawi, A.F.; Habib, S.L.; Mohammed, M.A.; Abadi, A.A.; Michael, M.S. Influence of cigarette smoking on prostaglandin synthesis and cyclooxygenase-2 gene expression in human urinary bladder cancer. *Cancer Investig.* **2002**, *20*, 651–656. [CrossRef]
15. Witjes, J.A.; Bruins, H.M.; Cathomas, R.; Compérat, E.M.; Cowan, N.C.; Gakis, G.; Hernández, V.; Espinós, E.E.; Lorch, A.; Neuzillet, Y.; et al. European Association of Urology Guidelines on Muscle-invasive and Metastatic Bladder Cancer: Summary of the 2020 Guidelines. *Eur. Urol.* **2021**, *79*, 82–104. [CrossRef]

Disclaimer/Publisher's Note: The statements, opinions and data contained in all publications are solely those of the individual author(s) and contributor(s) and not of MDPI and/or the editor(s). MDPI and/or the editor(s) disclaim responsibility for any injury to people or property resulting from any ideas, methods, instructions or products referred to in the content.

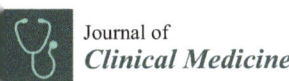

Article

Immunohistochemical Algorithm for the Classification of Muscle-Invasive Urinary Bladder Carcinoma with Lymph Node Metastasis: An Institutional Study

Karla Beatríz Peña [1,2,3], Francesc Riu [1,2,3], Josep Gumà [2,3,4], Francisca Martínez-Madueño [2,4], Maria José Miranda [2,4], Anna Vidal [2,4], Marc Grifoll [2,4], Joan Badia [2,4], Marta Rodriguez-Balada [2,4] and David Parada [1,2,3,*]

1. Molecular Pathology Unit, Department of Pathology, Hospital Universitari de Sant Joan, 43204 Reus, Spain
2. Institut d'Investigació Sanitària Pere Virgili, 43204 Reus, Spain
3. Facultat de Medicina i Ciències de la Salut, Universitat Rovira i Virgili, 43204 Reus, Spain
4. Institut d'Oncologia de la Catalunya Sud, Hospital Universitari Sant Joan de Reus, IISPV, URV, 43204 Reus, Spain
* Correspondence: david.parada@urv.cat

Abstract: Muscle-invasive urothelial carcinoma represents 20% of newly diagnosed cases of bladder cancer, and most cases show aggressive biological behavior with a poor prognosis. It is necessary to identify biomarkers that can be used as prognostic and predictive factors in daily clinical practice. In our study, we analyzed different antibodies in selected cases of muscle-invasive urinary bladder carcinoma and lymph node metastasis to identify immunohistochemical types and their value as possible prognostic factors. A total of 38 patients were included, 87% men and 13% women, with a mean age of 67.8 years. The most frequent histopathological type was urothelial carcinoma. In the primary lesion, the mixed type was the most common. In unilateral metastasis, the mixed type was the most frequently found. In cases of primary lesions and bilateral metastasis, the luminal and mixed types were observed. The luminal subtype was the most stable in immunohistochemical expression across primary tumors and metastases. The basal type showed a better prognosis in terms of disease-free survival. In conclusion, immunohistochemical studies are useful in assessing primary and metastatic lesions in patients with urothelial carcinoma. Immunohistochemical classification can typify muscle-invasive urothelial carcinoma, and the immunophenotype seems to have prognostic implications.

Keywords: bladder; cancer; muscle invasive; metastases; lymph node; immunohistochemical; classification; prognosis; heterogeneity

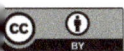

1. Introduction

Bladder cancer is the tenth most commonly diagnosed cancer worldwide, with approximately 573,000 new cases and 213,000 deaths per year [1,2]. The cancer is four times more frequent in men than in women and is the sixth most common cancer and ninth leading cause of cancer death among men [1,2]. Bladder cancer is a heterogeneous disease associated with diverse clinical outcomes. Thus, tumors that histologically invade the detrusor muscle are called muscle-invasive bladder cancers (MIBCs) and have a greater propensity to spread to lymph nodes and other organs [3–5]. When histologic examination shows no invasion into the detrusor muscle, then the cancer is termed nonmuscle invasive and comprises a variety of entities, including carcinoma in situ (CIS), noninvasive papillary tumors, and papillary tumors that invade the lamina propria [3–5].

MIBC accounts for approximately 20% of newly diagnosed cases of bladder cancer. Despite radical cystectomy (CR) and pelvic lymph node dissection, approximately 50% of patients will develop disease at distant sites due to disseminated micrometastases [6].

Urothelial carcinoma is the main tumor type, representing approximately 90% of neoplasms that affect the urinary bladder [2,7]. The epithelium from which urothelial carcinoma originates is the urothelium, which consists of stratified epithelium throughout the entire urinary system. Several studies have shown that the development of urothelial carcinoma may occur through two pathways, termed papillary and nonpapillary, leading to different but somewhat overlapping subsets of the disease with distinct molecular profiles [7–9]. In addition, tumor heterogeneity, both intertumoral and intratumoral, has been widely described [10,11], which makes it difficult to analyze both the primary and metastatic lesions of urothelial carcinoma.

Little is known about the variations in protein expression between primary bladder cancer and lymph node metastases. The aim of the present study was to compare the immunohistochemical (IHC) findings of patients with muscle-invasive urothelial carcinoma (MIUC) and lymph node metastases. In addition, the possibility of applying an IHC algorithm that allows for the classification of MIUC was evaluated. Finally, the prognostic value of the classification in patients with MIUC was investigated.

2. Materials and Methods

2.1. Patients

This retrospective and descriptive cohort study was performed in the MIUC of the urinary bladder patients who had undergone radical cystectomy and bilateral ileo-obturator lymphadenectomy. The study protocol was reviewed and approved by the Ethics Committee of the Sant Joan University Hospital in Reus (registration number CEIC11-04-28/4PROJ3), and written informed consent was obtained from each subject in accordance with the 1964 Helsinki Declaration and its subsequent amendments.

Thirty-eight patients with muscle invasive urothelial carcinoma who had undergone radical cystectomy and pelvic lymph node dissection were included from the Sant Joan University Hospital in Reus. The general criteria for patient selection were as follows: treated from January 2014 to January 2019; biopsy with a confirmed diagnosis of MIUC; uni- and/or bilateral lymph node metastases; absence of severe psychiatric disorders, chronic alcoholism or drug addiction; and adequate understanding of the surgery and adherence to follow-up standards. Patient charts were reviewed to collect data regarding sex, age at diagnosis, clinical stage, surgery, residual disease after surgery, systemic treatment, local recurrence, and survival.

2.2. Histopathological Study

The cystectomy specimens were opened through the urinary bladder and fixed in 10% buffered formalin for at least 48 h. After fixation, the biopsied sections from macroscopic lesions were embedded in paraffin, cut into 2 μm sections, and stained with hematoxylin and eosin (H&E). All dissected lymph node material was embedded in paraffin and prepared following the previous staining protocol. For each case of radical cystectomy, tumor histology, grade (according to the 2022 World Health Organization) [12], pathological stage, presence of carcinoma in situ (CIS), lymphovascular invasion, and margin status were analyzed. In cases of lymph node dissection, the total number of lymph nodes, number of metastatic lymph nodes, size of large metastases, and extra-capsular lymph node involvement were evaluated.

2.3. Immunohistochemical Study

Two-micrometer sections were obtained from both paraffin-embedded MIUC and lymph node metastases samples and were placed in a VENTANA® Benchmark UL-TRA/LT immunohistochemistry automatic processor, Ventana Medical Systems, USA, using the standardized protocol for uroplakin, GATA3, cytokeratin 5, cytokeratin 14, cytokeratin 18, cytokeratin 20, and CD44, including retrieval solution, pH 9, and a detection kit for Immunohistochemistry Optiview® DAB (VENTANA®). The primary anti-uroplakin, GATA3, cytokeratin 5, cytokeratin 14, cytokeratin 18, cytokeratin 20, and CD44 antibodies (prediluted) (Phoenix Pharmaceutical, Inc.) were incubated for 32 min. Finally, the IHC sections were revealed with diaminobenzidine, contrasted with Meyer's hematoxylin, and examined under an Olympus BX41 light microscope, with direct in-creases in magnification ranging from 2× to 60×. The IHC images of both MIUC and lymph node metastases were evaluated by two independent pathologists.

2.4. Semiquantitative Evaluation of Immunoreactivity

IHC interpretation was performed using combined intensity and percentage scales defined by different groups to assess IHC profiles [8,13–15]. All tumor areas of both MIUC and lymph node metastases were evaluated. Positive IHC staining for an antibody was considered when cytoplasmic or nuclear staining was observed, depending on the antibody tested. Each antibody was assigned a percentage of positivity, with the following positivity intervals: 0% as negative, between 1 to 10%, between 11 to 50%, between 51 to 80%, and greater than 80%. Additionally, intense cytoplasmatic IHC staining was scored as follows: negative: no staining; 1+: weak staining; 2+: moderate staining, and 3+: intense staining. Appropriate positive and negative controls were used for each antibody. Additionally, the reactivity of the positive controls served to assess the intensity of the staining. The magnification varied between 4×, 10× and 20×.

2.5. Statistical Analysis

Descriptive statistics are presented as N (%) for qualitative clinical variables, while median, 25th percentile (P25) and 75th percentile (P75) are used for quantitative clinical variables. Statistical analyses were carried out in R (version 4.2.0).

Hierarchical clustering was performed on the immunohistochemistry (IHC) antibody expression in bladder tissue using the pvclust R package (version 2.2-0) with default settings, which allowed us to assess the robustness of each cluster by bootstrapping with resampling (nboot = 1000). The clusters with an approximate unbiased (AU) p value ≥ 95 were deemed statistically significant (significance level < 0.05) and used in survival analysis, while samples not robustly assigned to any cluster (unassigned) were excluded from survival analysis. The clusters were then labeled according to CK20 and CK18 bladder tissue expression as luminal, basal or mixed type and according to CK5 and GATA bladder tissue expression as CK5± or GATA± subtypes. Heatmaps of IHC antibody expression were generated with the ComplexHeatmap R package (version 2.12.0) using the dendrogram from bootstrap hierarchical clustering (top dendrogram).

Survival analysis was performed with the survival (version 3.3-1) and survminer R packages (version 0.4.9). Progression-free survival (PFS) is defined as the time from cystectomy surgery until a detected progression according to the Response Evaluation Criteria in Solid Tumors (RECIST) or date of last contact (right-censored point). Overall survival was defined as the time from cystectomy surgery until a known death event or date of last contact (right-censored point).

The suggested algorithm for MIBC subtype classification included a 20% expression cutoff. Alternative cutoffs are also represented for each cluster.

3. Results

3.1. Clinical Findings

A total of 38 patients were included in the study, comprising 33 (87%) men and 5 (13%) women, with a mean age of 67.8 years (62–75 years). The most frequent pathological stage (pT) was T3 in 18 patients (50%), followed by T4 in 15 patients (40%) and finally stage T2 in 4 patients (10%). Cystectomy was the only initial treatment in 30 patients (79%), in the other 8 of the 38 included patients received a combined treatment of cystectomy and chemotherapy (CT) (4 patients, 11%), cystectomy plus immunotherapy (IT) (2 patients, 5%), combination of cystectomy plus chemotherapy and immunotherapy (1 patient, 3%) and surgical treatment plus radiotherapy (RT) (1 patient, 3%). A total of 18 patients

(47%) showed progression of urothelial carcinoma, and 24 patients (63%) died of bladder carcinoma. Table 1 summarizes the clinical findings.

Table 1. Clinical findings in patients with muscle-invasive urinary bladder carcinoma and lymph node metastases ($n = 38$).

	Urothelial	Urothelial Combined	Others	All
	$n = 14$	$n = 14$	$n = 10$	$n = 38$
Age				
Mean	68.4 years	68.2 years	66.4 years	67.8 years
Median (P25, P75)	66.5 (63, 77)	69.5 (63, 73)	65.5 (59, 73)	67.5 (62, 75)
Sex				
Men	13 (93%)	12 (86%)	8 (80%)	33 (87%)
Women	1 (7%)	2 (14%)	2 (20%)	5 (13%)
Stage				
pT2	1 (7%)	2 (14%)	1 (10%)	4 (10%)
pT3	5 (36%)	7 (50%)	7 (70%)	18 (50%)
pT4	8 (57%)	5 (36%)	2 (20%)	15 (40%)
Unilateral or bilateral pelvic lymph node metastases				
Unilateral (NT1)	10 (71%)	9 (64%)	4 (40%)	23 (61%)
Bilateral (NT2)	4 (29%)	5 (36%)	6 (60%)	15 (39%)
Distant metastases				
M0	9 (64%)	14 (100%)	9 (90%)	32 (84%)
M1	5 (36%)	0	1 (10%)	6 (16%)
Morphology				
Pure urothelial	14 (100%)	0	0	14 (37%)
Urothelial + squamous	0	7 (50%)	0	7 (18%)
Pure squamous	0	0	5 (50%)	5 (13%)
Others	0	7 (50%)	5 (50%)	12 (32%)
Primary treatment				
Only cystectomy	10 (71%)	11 (79%)	9 (90%)	30 (79%)
Cystectomy + CT	2 (14%)	1 (7%)	1 (10%)	4 (11%)
Cystectomy + IT	1 (7%)	1 (7%)	0	2 (5%)
Cystectomy + CT + IT	1 (7%)	0	0	1 (3%)
Cystectomy + RT	0	1 (7%)	0	1 (3%)
Adjuvant chemotherapy				
N (%)	5 (36%)	11 (79%)	4 (40%)	20 (53%)
Progression				
N (%)	5 (36%)	6 (43%)	2 (20%)	13 (34%)
Death				
N (%)	9 (64%)	8 (57%)	6 (60%)	23 (61%)

Abbreviations: CT = chemotherapy; IT = immunotherapy; RT = radiotherapy; SD = standard deviation Q25 = quartile 25; Q75 = quartile 75.

3.2. Histopathological Findings

Urothelial carcinoma was the most frequent histological type, found in 14 tumors (37%), followed by urothelial carcinoma with divergent squamous differentiation in 7 tumors (18%). Five tumors (13%) were pure squamous cell carcinomas, and 12 carcinomas (32%) showed combinations of different histological types of carcinomas, such as solid urothelial carcinoma with micropapillary carcinoma, sarcomatoid urothelial carcinoma, urothelial carcinoma with glycogen-rich carcinoma, and urothelial carcinoma with plasmacytoid carcinoma (Figure 1). The histopathological study of the pelvic lymph node dissection samples showed that between 1 and 25 lymph nodes (mean: 7.86) were evaluated in right lymphadenectomy and between 1 and 20 lymph nodes (mean: 8.53) were evaluated in left lymphadenectomy. In total, 23 (60.53%) patients showed unilateral lymph node metastasis, 11 patients out of 23 showed lymph node metastasis on only the right side (1–3 metastatic nodes, mean: 1.64), and in the remaining 12 patients, only the left side was affected (1–3 metastatic nodes, mean: 1.92). In 15 patients (39.47%), bilateral lymph node metastasis was observed (1–17 metastatic lymph nodes, mean: 4.24).

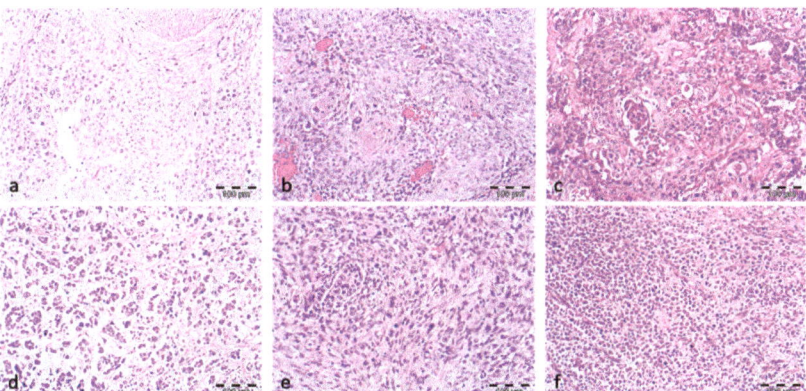

Figure 1. Histopathological findings of muscle-invasive urothelial cell carcinoma. (**a**) Urothelial cell carcinoma. (**b**) Urothelial cell carcinoma with divergent squamous differentiation. (**c**) Pure squamous cell carcinoma. (**d**) Micropapillary carcinoma. (**e**) Sarcomatoid carcinoma. (**f**) Plasmacytoid carcinoma. (HE, 10×).

3.3. Immunohistochemical Findings

3.3.1. Muscle-Invasive Urothelial Carcinoma

The IHC study showed that GATA3 was the most frequently expressed marker, in 94.74% of the patients, followed by cytokeratin 18 (92.11%) and cytokeratin 5 (89.47%). Uroplakin was expressed in 26.32% of the patients. The immunoreaction intensity ranged from 2+ to 3+, and the percentage of positive cells ranged from 1% to 90%. In general, the expression of basal markers (CK5, CK14 and CD44) was seen in 68.51% of the patients, while luminal markers (uroplakin, CK20, and CK18) were demonstrated in 55.27% of the patients (Figure 2).

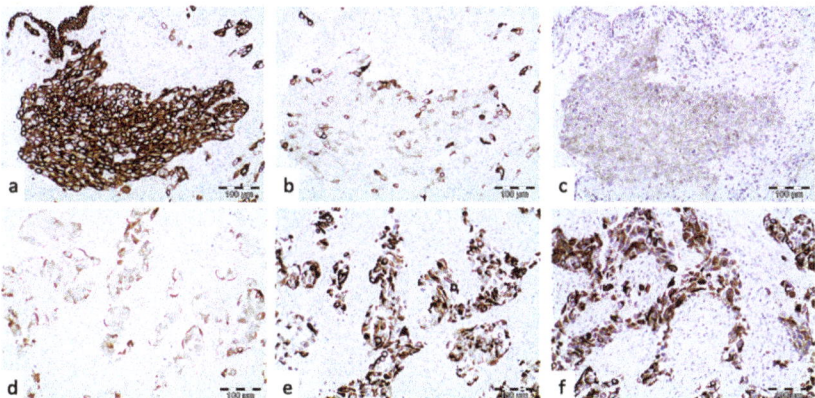

Figure 2. Inmunohistological findings in muscle-invasive urothelial cell carcinoma basal markers (**a–c**). (**a**) Diffuse and strong expression of cytokeratin is shown. (**b**) Cytokeratin 14 showing focal cytoplasmic positivity. (**c**) CD44 cytoplasmic expression in neoplastic urothelial cells. Luminal markers (**d–f**). (**d**) Uroplaquin showing cytoplasmic positivity in neoplastic cells. (**e**) Neoplastic cells with cytoplasmic cytokeratin 20 expression. (**f**) Diffuse and intensive cytoplasmic expression of cytokeratin 18 is shown. (Diaminobenzidine (DAB), 10×).

To try to define specific clusters that would facilitate defining specific subtypes of urothelial carcinoma, the bootstrap clustering algorithm ($n = 1000$) was applied and showed clusters with significant differences between groups ($p < 0.05$). Subsequently, heatmap analysis was able to identify basal and luminal groups based on the expression of luminal markers, such as cytokeratin 20 and cytokeratin 18 or on the expression of basal markers, such as cytokeratin 5 and 14. Cluster 5 showed ex-pression of luminal markers and basal markers (cytokeratin 18 and cytokeratin 5) and was considered a mixed immunophenotype. Finally, cluster 6 showed a loss of cytokeratin 20 despite expressing cytokeratin 10 (Figure 3).

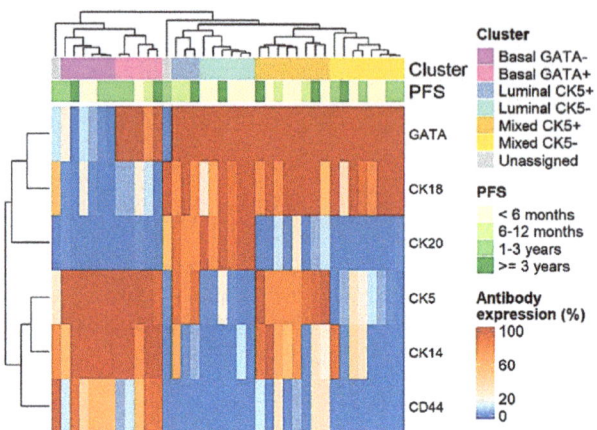

Figure 3. Heatmap of antibody expression (%). Hierarchical clustering with bootstrapping identified 6 clusters, which were labeled luminal, basal or mixed according to the expression of the markers CK20 and CK18. Luminal clusters expressed both markers, mixed clusters expressed only CK18, while basal clusters lacked both markers. Clusters were then further subdivided and labeled according to the expression of CK5 or GATA.

Based on the results obtained in bootstrap clustering and heatmap analysis, the following algorithm was proposed for the classification of MIUCs (Figure 4), with a cutoff of 20% for each antibody analyzed (Figures 4 and 5):

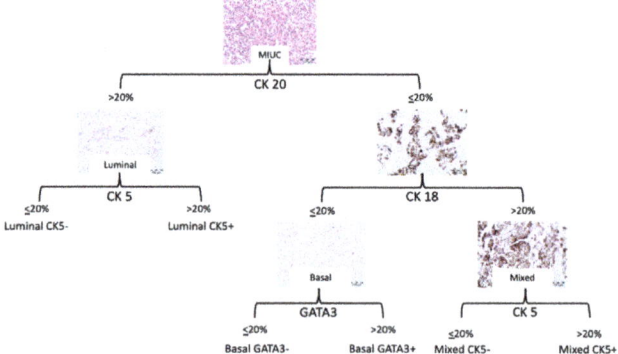

Figure 4. Proposed algorithm based on two markers and the representation of the bootstrap clustering results and heatmap analysis.

By applying the algorithm based on two markers for MIUCs, it was possible to classify 11 patients (28.95%) as having a luminal immunophenotype, 10 patients (26.32%) as having a basal immunophenotype, and 16 patients (42.11%) as having a mixed immunophenotype. One patient (2.63%) could not be classified with a morphology that corresponded to urothelial carcinoma with divergent squamous differentiation and a plasmacytoid carcinoma component.

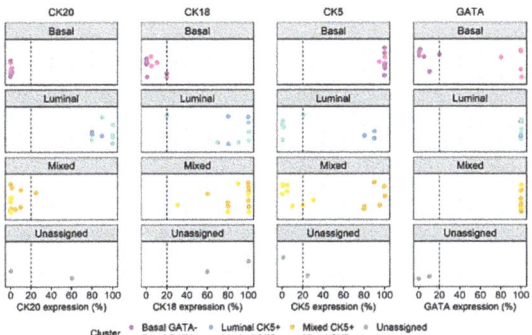

Figure 5. Antibody expression showing the 20% cutoff (dotted vertical line) for each cluster.

3.3.2. Unilateral Pelvic Lymph Node Metastasis

In general, the immunohistochemical study showed that GATA3 was the most frequently expressed marker in 86.96% of metastatic pelvic lymph nodes, followed by cytokeratin 5 (91.30%), and cytokeratin 18 (88.96%). Uroplakin was evidenced in 20.09%. The immunoreaction intensity was from 2+ to 3+, and the percentage of positive cells varied between 1% to 90. The expression of basal markers (CK5, CK14 and CD44) was evidenced in 62.32% of the patients, while luminal markers (uroplakin, CK20, and CK18) were demonstrated in 54.96% of cases. Applying the algorithm of 2 markers pelvic lymph node metastatic carcinomas could be classified in 14 patients (36.84%) as luminal immunophenotype, 8 patients (21.05%) as basal immunophenotype, and 16 patients (42.11%) were classified as mixed immunophenotype.

3.3.3. Bilateral Pelvic Lymph Node Metastasis

In patients with bilateral pelvic lymph node metastases, GATA3 could be observed in 93.33% and 100% of the two regions analyzed, followed by cytokeratin 18 (100% of the two regions) and cytokeratin 5 (86.67% of the two regions). Cytokeratin 20 was detected in 66.67% and 80% of patients, cytokeratin 14 in 60% and 33.33%, CD44 in 33.33% and 26.67%, and uroplakin in 26.67% and 40%. When the cases were analyzed in pairs ($n = 15$), the expression of basal markers (CK5, CK14 and CD44) was observed in 60% and 48.89% of each region studied, while the expression of luminal markers (uroplakin, CK20, and CK18) was demonstrated in 64.45% and 73.33% of the cases according to each region analyzed. Eight lymph node metastases (53.33%) were classified as having a luminal immunophenotype, and the remaining seven lymph node metastases (46.67%) were classified as having a mixed immunophenotype.

3.3.4. Urothelial Carcinoma and Unilateral Pelvic Lymph Node Metastasis

Using the immunophenotype classification algorithm, it was possible to show that in the 11 patients with a luminal immunophenotype, 10 maintained this immunophenotype in the pelvic lymph node metastases (90.91%), and the remaining patient (9.09%) showed a basal immunophenotype in the pelvic lymph node metastasis. Overall, the baseline primary immunophenotype (10 patients) remained the same immunophenotype in 6 patients (60%), while the immunophenotype became mixed in 3 patients (30%) and luminal in 1 patient (10%). The mixed primary immunophenotype (16) was seen in the lymph node metastases of 12 patients (75%); 3 metastatic carcinomas (18.75%) were classified as luminal; and 1 carcinoma (6.25%) was classified as basal. The patient whose primary bladder lesion could not be classified showed a mixed immunophenotype in the pelvic lymph node metastasis.

3.3.5. Urothelial Carcinoma and Bilateral Pelvic Lymph Node Metastasis (Paired Cases)

In the 15 patients with bilateral pelvic lymph node metastasis, the immunophenotype classification algorithm was able to show that in the 6 patients with luminal immunophenotype 5 and 6, the immunophenotype maintained in the pelvic lymph node metastases.

Overall, the primary basal immunophenotype observed in the two primary lesions were basal in one lesion and mixed in one of the metastases, and on the contralateral side, the immunophenotype was mixed in both. The primary mixed immunophenotype (6) was evidenced in the pelvic lymph node metastases of 4 patients (75%), and the remaining two metastases were luminal; among the contralateral metastases, five were classified as mixed, and the remaining 3 were classified as luminal.

Kaplan–Meier analysis for PFS was performed in the immunohistochemistry (IHC) groups. The IHC groups suggested a significant association between group identity and the PFS rate. Specifically, the luminal and basal clusters from the identified seven-marker expression cluster were significantly associated with PFS rate. Kaplan-Meier analysis for PFS was also performed to assess the simplified two-marker algorithm, which could nearly replicate the resulting bootstrap clusters and also showed a significant association with PFS rate (Figure 6a,b). No significant differences were observed between unilateral and bilateral pelvic lymph node metastases (Figures 6 and 7).

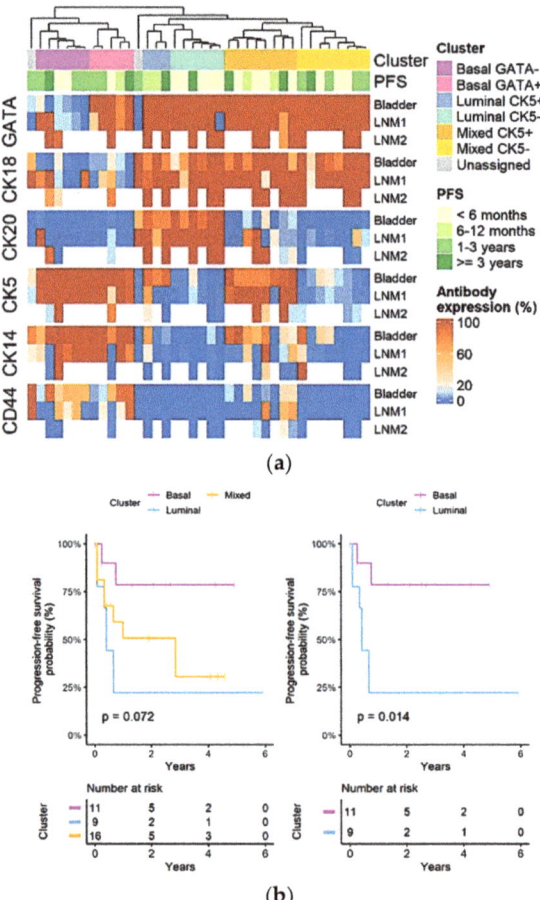

Figure 6. Heatmap of antibody expression (%) for bladder and pelvic lymph node metastasis tissues (**a**). Survival analysis of IHC clusters suggested a significant association between cluster identity and progression-free survival (PFS) rate. Specifically, luminal and basal IHC clusters were significantly associated with PFS rates (**b**).

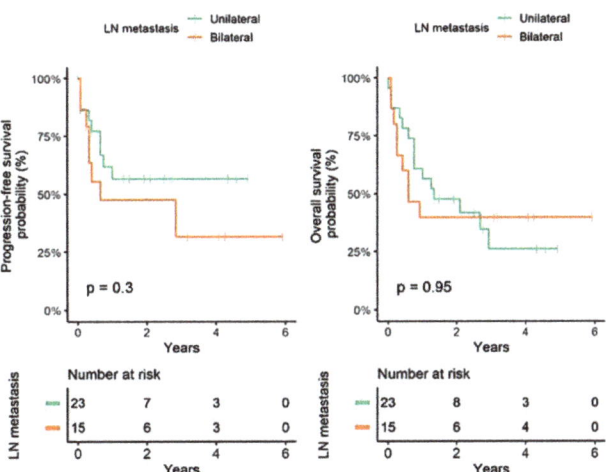

Figure 7. Survival analysis for unilateral or bilateral pelvic lymph node metastasis.

4. Discussion

Invasive urothelial carcinoma is the most common malignant neoplasm of the urinary tract. MIUCs represent approximately 20–25% of all cancers in the urinary bladder [16], and most of them show rapid progression and metastasis and are associated with a poor prognosis. In the present study, we analyzed a series of patients who underwent radical cystectomy for a diagnosis of MIUC, showing cancer progression in 47% of patients and a cancer-specific mortality rate of 63%. In addition, all patients evaluated had lymph node metastases, which may negatively affect the outcome [17]. Our findings support that MIUC is an aggressive neoplasm with a poor prognosis, and it is necessary to identify new markers that can be used as prognostic and predictive factors in this cancer.

Bladder cancer is often histologically heterogeneous within a given patient. This is well demonstrated by the frequent coexistence of conventional urothelial carcinoma and named histologic variants of bladder cancer, such as squamous and micropapillary cancers [11]. In the present study, the histopathological heterogeneity in MIBC was confirmed, since approximately 50% of the cancers evaluated were urothelial carcinoma with a divergent squamous differentiation and a combination of morphological variants, including more aggressive variants, such as micropapillary carcinoma, sarcomatoid carcinoma, and plasmacytoid carcinoma [18,19]. An interesting finding was that five patients who were diagnosed after extensive pathologic examination of the carcinoma had pure squamous cell carcinoma, without evidence of a urothelial carcinoma component. This finding represents a three times higher rate of pure squamous cell carcinoma than the reported incidence and could be related to the possible etiological factors associated with this cancer, such as smoking, since these patients had a higher intensity of smoking [12]. The recent classification of tumors of the genitourinary system of 2022 noted the importance of reporting the different components of conventional urothelial carcinoma, as well as the histological subtypes and the divergent differentiation in each tumor. The need to quantify these elements was also indicated, given their possible implications for patient management [19].

Tumor heterogeneity in MIUC, in addition to morphological variability, also includes diversity from a molecular point of view [19,20]. This molecular diversity implies different omic expressions [21], such as at the protein level. The study of protein expression has made it possible to discover different cellular components in the urothelium, which has facilitated the characterization of umbrella cells, superficial cells, intermediate cells and basal cells [22]. In addition, this knowledge has made it possible to establish the dual-track concept of bladder carcinogenesis [7]. This concept suggests that parabasal cells give rise to superficial papillary lesions through the papillary luminal pathway, while basal cells that progress through the nonpapillary basal pathway give rise to invasive lesions [7]. In the present study, we demonstrated variable expression of both luminal and basal markers in MIUC, with a higher expression of basal markers. This finding differs from that reported by other studies in which MIUC was analyzed by whole-transcriptome mRNA expression profiling, and the luminal type was found to be the most frequent, followed by the basal and double negative subtypes [23]. However, from an IHC point of view, our findings confirm the heterogeneity of protein expression in this type of cancer and that invasive lesions, in general, express markers related to the nonpapillary basal pathway.

In the present study, to develop a potential IHC classifier of molecular subtypes of MIBC and lymph node metastasis that can be used in routine clinical practice, we analyzed 7 previously described markers [7,13–15]. Our analysis showed that cytokeratin 20 and cytokeratin 18 are the two markers that enabled differentiation between the luminal and basal subtypes. In addition, our study confirmed the usefulness of the 20% cutoff point to interpret the positivity of the investigated markers, showing coincident results with those published by other studies on the expression of basal and luminal markers in urothelial carcinoma [8,15]. In addition, the classification of subtypes in MIUC in our study showed significant differences in overall survival between the groups analyzed, with a worse prognosis for the luminal subtype than for the basal and mixed subtypes. This finding differs from what has been shown in other studies in which the basal subtype was associated with a worse prognosis [24]; however, other researchers have not shown differences in DSS or other clinical prognostic factors suggesting a better prognosis for the basal subtype, even though the results showed trends without statistical significance [25]. A possible explanation for this difference is that we included patients with advanced stages and lymph node metastasis, which requires therapeutic interventions. This may imply that basal tumors respond better to these therapies. Another factor that could affect this difference is the expression of genes related to tumor metabolism, which would imply differences in immunotherapy response, as well as variable responses to cisplatin, doxorubicin, and other first-line anticancer drugs [26].

Another aspect of our study consisted of studying the evolution of the expression of IHC markers, comparing bladder tumors and lymph node metastases. The relationship between the primary tumor and unilateral lymph node metastasis showed that the luminal immunophenotype was the most stable, since in bladder carcinomas with this immunophenotype, 90% showed the same luminal type in the unilateral lymph node metastases, and only one case showed a basal immunophenotype. On the other hand, the basal type maintained its immunophenotype in 60% of the unilateral lymph node metastases and changed to luminal and mixed immunophenotypes in the rest of the patients. Finally, the mixed immunophenotype persisted in 75% of the patients, showing basal and luminal immunophenotypes in the rest of the patients. Sjödahl et al. [27] studied MIUC and lymph node metastases using immunohistochemistry and gene expression profiling, and they showed that the basal/squamous-like subtype was the most discordant type. Our results confirm that the basal and mixed immunophenotypes are the most discordant in terms of immunohistochemistry and demonstrate the IHC plasticity of both immunophenotypes, while the luminal type was more stable in terms of its immunophenotypic expression in patients with unilateral lymph node metastasis. In patients with bilateral lymph node metastases (paired cases), the immunophenotypic variations were greater in one of the two metastatic regions evaluated. In general, the basal immunophenotype was not found in one of the metastatic regions, while the luminal and mixed immunophenotypes persisted in lymph node metastases. Further studies are necessary to try to understand the significance of the immunophenotypic variations among MIUC, unilateral and/or bilateral metastases and the prognostic and predictive role of these variations in these patients.

Our study has some limitations, such as the low number of patients included in the study, although our sample comprises a particular group of patients with MIUC and lymph node metastasis. Additionally, the imaging study was carried out semi-quantitatively;

however, this analysis represents a useful tool in daily clinical practice and can serve as a basis for using specialized tools for quantitative image analysis.

5. Conclusions

In summary, our study demonstrated that MIUC represents a heterogeneous disease at different stages, with fundamental clinical implications for its prognosis and serves as the basis for possible predictive factors. The IHC study was a useful tool to assess primary and metastatic lesions in patients with urothelial carcinoma, and by applying a classification system based on two markers, the different subtypes of MIUC could be typified. The classification of the different subtypes seems to have prognostic implications and could help to stratify patients.

Author Contributions: Conceptualization, D.P.; methodology, D.P. and K.B.P.; validation, D.P., K.B.P. and J.B.; formal analysis, D.P. and J.B.; investigation, D.P., F.M.-M., M.J.M., A.V., F.R. and J.G.; resources, D.P. and F.R.; data curation, D.P., J.B., M.G., M.R.-B. and J.G.; writing—original draft preparation, D.P.; writing—review and editing, D.P.; visualization, D.P.; supervision, D.P. All authors have read and agreed to the published version of the manuscript.

Funding: This research received no external funding.

Institutional Review Board Statement: The study was conducted in accordance with the Declaration of Helsinki and approved by the Ethics Committee of the Sant Joan University Hospital in Reus (registration number CEIC11-04-28/4PROJ3) for studies involving humans.

Informed Consent Statement: Informed consent was obtained from all subjects involved in the study.

Data Availability Statement: All of the data are present in the manuscript.

Conflicts of Interest: The authors declare no conflict of interest.

References

1. Sung, H.; Ferlay, J.; Siegel, R.L.; Laversanne, M.; Soerjomataram, I.; Jemal, A.; Bray, F. Global Cancer Statistics 2020: GLOBOCAN Estimates of Incidence and Mortality Worldwide for 36 Cancers in 185 Countries. *CA Cancer J. Clin.* **2021**, *71*, 209–249. [CrossRef] [PubMed]
2. Siegel, R.L.; Miller, K.D.; Fuchs, H.E.; Jemal, A. Cancer statistics, 2022. *CA Cancer J. Clin.* **2022**, *72*, 7–33. [CrossRef] [PubMed]
3. Dinney, C.P.; McConkey, D.J.; Millikan, R.E.; Wu, X.; Bar-Eli, M.; Adam, L.; Kamat, A.M.; Siefker-Radtke, A.O.; Tuziak, T.; Sabichi, A.L.; et al. Focus on bladder cancer. *Cancer Cell* **2004**, *6*, 111–116. [CrossRef] [PubMed]
4. Kamat, A.M.; Hahn, N.M.; Efstathiou, J.A.; Lerner, S.P.; Malmström, P.U.; Choi, W.; Guo, C.C.; Lotan, Y.; Kassouf, W. Bladder cancer. *Lancet* **2016**, *3*, 2796–2810. [CrossRef]
5. Knowles, M.A.; Hurst, C.D. Molecular biology of bladder cancer: New insights into pathogenesis and clinical diversity. *Nat. Rev. Cancer* **2015**, *15*, 25–41. [CrossRef]
6. Patel, V.G.; Oh, W.K.; Galsky, M.D. Treatment of muscle-invasive and advanced bladder cancer in 2020. *CA Cancer J. Clin.* **2020**, *70*, 404–423. [CrossRef]
7. Guo, C.C.; Czerniak, B. Bladder Cancer in the Genomic Era. *Arch. Pathol. Lab. Med.* **2019**, *143*, 695–704. [CrossRef]
8. Dadhania, V.; Zhang, M.; Zhang, L.; Bondaruk, J.; Majewski, T.; Siefker-Radtke, A.; Guo, C.C.; Dinney, C.; Cogdell, D.E.; Zhang, S.; et al. Meta-Analysis of the Luminal and Basal Subtypes of Bladder Cancer and the Identification of Signature Immunohistochemical Markers for Clinical Use. *EBioMedicine* **2016**, *12*, 105–117. [CrossRef]
9. Kamoun, A.; de Reyniès, A.; Allory, Y.; Sjödahl, G.; Robertson, A.G.; Seiler, R.; Hoadley, K.A.; Groeneveld, C.S.; Al-Ahmadie, H.; Bladder Cancer Molecular Taxonomy Group; et al. A Consensus Molecular Classification of Muscle-invasive Bladder Cancer. *Eur. Urol.* **2020**, *77*, 420–433. [CrossRef]
10. da Costa, J.B.; Gibb, E.A.; Nykopp, T.K.; Mannas, M.; Wyatt, A.W.; Black, P.C. Molecular tumor heterogeneity in muscle invasive bladder cancer: Biomarkers, subtypes, and implications for therapy. *Urol. Oncol.* **2022**, *40*, 287–294. [CrossRef]
11. Warrick, J.I.; Sjödahl, G.; Kaag, M.; Raman, J.D.; Merrill, S.; Shuman, L.; Chen, G.; Walter, V.; DeGraff, D.J. Intratumoral Heterogeneity of Bladder Cancer by Molecular Subtypes and Histologic Variants. *Eur. Urol.* **2019**, *75*, 18–22. [CrossRef] [PubMed]
12. WHO. *Classification of Tumours of the Urinary System and Male Genital Organs*, 5th ed.; International Agency for Research on Cancer: Lyon, France, 2022.
13. Johnson, S.M.; Khararjian, A.; Legesse, T.B.; Khani, F.; Robinson, B.D.; Epstein, J.I.; Wobker, S.E. Nested Variant of Urothelial Carcinoma Is a Luminal Bladder Tumor with Distinct Coexpression of the Basal Marker Cytokeratin 5/6. *Am. J. Clin. Pathol.* **2021**, *155*, 588–596. [CrossRef] [PubMed]

14. Weyerer, V.; Weisser, R.; Moskalev, E.A.; Haller, F.; Stoehr, R.; Eckstein, M.; Zinnall, U.; Gaisa, N.T.; Compérat, E.; Perren, A.; et al. Distinct genetic alterations and luminal molecular subtype in nested variant of urothelial carcinoma. *Histopathology* **2019**, *75*, 865–875. [CrossRef] [PubMed]
15. Hodgson, A.; Liu, S.K.; Vesprini, D.; Xu, B.; Downes, M.R. Basal-subtype bladder tumours show a 'hot' immunophenotype. *Histopathology* **2018**, *73*, 748–757. [CrossRef]
16. AZhaTi, B.; Wu, G.; Zhan, H.; Liang, W.; Song, Z.; Lu, L.; Xie, Q. Alternative splicing patterns reveal prognostic indicator in muscle-invasive bladder cancer. *World J. Surg. Oncol.* **2022**, *20*, 231. [CrossRef]
17. Koppie, T.M.; Vickers, A.J.; Vora, K.; Dalbagni, G.; Bochner, B.H. Standardization of pelvic lymphadenectomy performed at radical cystectomy: Can we establish a minimum number of lymph nodes that should be removed? *Cancer* **2006**, *107*, 2368–2374. [CrossRef]
18. Lopez-Beltran, A.; Henriques, V.; Montironi, R.; Cimadamore, A.; Raspollini, M.R.; Cheng, L. Variants and new entities of bladder cancer. *Histopathology* **2019**, *74*, 77–96. [CrossRef]
19. Netto, G.J.; Amin, M.B.; Berney, D.M.; Compérat, E.M.; Gill, A.J.; Hartmann, A.; Menon, S.; Raspollini, M.R.; Rubin, M.A.; Srigley, J.R.; et al. The 2022 World Health Organization Classification of Tumors of the Urinary System and Male Genital Organs-Part B: Prostate and Urinary Tract Tumors. *Eur. Urol.* **2022**, *82*, 469–482. [CrossRef]
20. Choi, W.; Porten, S.; Kim, S.; Willis, D.; Plimack, E.R.; Hoffman-Censits, J.; Roth, B.; Cheng, T.; Tran, M.; Lee, I.L.; et al. Identification of distinct basal and luminal subtypes of muscle-invasive bladder cancer with different sensitivities to frontline chemotherapy. *Cancer Cell* **2014**, *25*, 152–165. [CrossRef]
21. Lindskrog, S.V.; Prip, F.; Lamy, P.; Taber, A.; Groeneveld, C.S.; Birkenkamp-Demtröder, K.; Jensen, J.B.; Strandgaard, T.; Nordentoft, I.; Christensen, E.; et al. An integrated multi-omics analysis identifies prognostic molecular subtypes of non-muscle-invasive bladder cancer. *Nat. Commun.* **2021**, *12*, 2301. [CrossRef]
22. López-Cortés, R.; Vázquez-Estévez, S.; Fernández, J.Á.; Núñez, C. Proteomics as a Complementary Technique to Characterize Bladder Cancer. *Cancers* **2021**, *13*, 5537. [CrossRef] [PubMed]
23. Guo, C.C.; Bondaruk, J.; Yao, H.; Wang, Z.; Zhang, L.; Lee, S.; Lee, J.G.; Cogdell, D.; Zhang, M.; Yang, G.; et al. Assessment of Luminal and Basal Phenotypes in Bladder Cancer. *Sci. Rep.* **2020**, *10*, 9743. [CrossRef] [PubMed]
24. Rodriguez Pena, M.; Chaux, A.; Eich, M.L.; Tregnago, A.C.; Taheri, D.; Borhan, W.; Sharma, R.; Rezaei, M.K.; Netto, G.J. Immunohistochemical assessment of basal and luminal markers in non-muscle invasive urothelial carcinoma of bladder. *Virch. Arch.* **2019**, *475*, 349–356. [CrossRef]
25. Weyerer, V.; Stoehr, R.; Bertz, S.; Lange, F.; Geppert, C.I.; Wach, S.; Taubert, H.; Sikic, D.; Wullich, B.; Hartmann, A.; et al. Prognostic impact of molecular muscle-invasive bladder cancer subtyping approaches and correlations with variant histology in a population-based mono-institutional cystectomy cohort. *World J. Urol.* **2021**, *39*, 4011–4019. [CrossRef] [PubMed]
26. Tang, C.; Yu, M.; Ma, J.; Zhu, Y. Metabolic classification of bladder cancer based on multi-omics integrated analysis to predict patient prognosis and treatment response. *J. Transl. Med.* **2021**, *19*, 205. [CrossRef]
27. Sjödahl, G.; Eriksson, P.; Lövgren, K.; Marzouka, N.A.; Bernardo, C.; Nordentoft, I.; Dyrskjøt, L.; Liedberg, F.; Höglund, M. Discordant molecular subtype classification in the basal-squamous subtype of bladder tumors and matched lymph-node metastases. *Mod. Pathol.* **2018**, *31*, 1869–1881. [CrossRef]

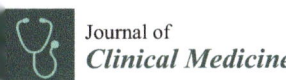

Article

Prognostic Utility of the Modified Glasgow Prognostic Score in Urothelial Carcinoma: Outcomes from a Pooled Analysis

Daqing Tan [1,2,†], Jinze Li [1,†], Tianhai Lin [1], Ping Tan [1], Jiapeng Zhang [1], Qiao Xiong [1], Jinjiang Jiang [1], Yifan Li [1], Peng Zhang [1,*] and Qiang Wei [1,*]

1. Department of Urology, Institute of Urology, West China Hospital, Sichuan University, Chengdu 610041, China
2. Department of Urology, Minda Hospital of Hubei Minzu University, Enshi 445000, China
* Correspondence: zpeng2001@163.com (P.Z.); weiqiang933@126.com (Q.W.)
† These authors contributed equally to this work.

Abstract: Background: Many studies explored the prognostic value of the modified Glasgow Prognostic Score (mGPS) in urothelial carcinoma (UC), but the results are controversial. This study aimed to quantify the relationship between pretreatment mGPS and survival in patients with UC. Methods: A systematic literature search was conducted using Embase, PubMed, and Web of Science to identify eligible studies published before August 2022. Pooled hazard ratios (HRs) with 95% confidence intervals (CIs) were used to assess the association between pretreatment mGPS and the prognosis of UC. Results: Thirteen eligible studies involving 12,524 patients were included. A high mGPS was significantly associated with poor overall survival (mGPS 1/0: HR = 1.33, 95% CI 1.12–1.58, $p = 0.001$; mGPS 2/0: HR = 2.02, 95% CI 1.43–2.84, $p < 0.0001$), progression-free survival (mGPS 1/0: HR = 1.26, 95% CI 1.03–1.53, $p = 0.021$; mGPS 2/0: HR = 1.76, 95% CI 1.12–2.77, $p = 0.013$), recurrence-free survival (mGPS 1/0: HR = 1.36, 95% CI 1.18–1.56, $p < 0.0001$; mGPS 2/0: HR = 1.70, 95% CI 1.44–2.000, $p < 0.0001$), and cancer-specific survival (mGPS 2/0: HR = 1.81, 95% CI 1.30–2.52, $p < 0.0001$). A subgroup analysis of OS also yielded similar results. Conclusions: Evidence suggests that high pretreatment mGPS in UC is closely related to poor survival. Pre-treatment mGPS is a powerful independent prognostic factor in patients with UC.

Keywords: modified Glasgow Prognostic Score; urothelial carcinoma; prognosis; survival; meta-analysis

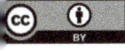

1. Introduction

Urothelial carcinoma (UC), including bladder cancer (BC) and upper urinary tract urothelial carcinoma (UTUC), is a common tumor of the urinary system. More than 90% of bladder cancer is histologically classified as UC [1]. UTUC is relatively rare, accounting for only 5–10% of all UCs [2]. Due to the multifocal nature of UC throughout the entire urinary tract (synchronously or metachronously), the 5-year survival rate is only 50% even after radical resection of BC, and 15–50% of UTUC patients undergoing surgical treatment experience recurrence during follow-up [3–5]. Therefore, a simple and accurate indicator is urgently needed for the early detection and identification of progression or prognosis in patients with UC.

The current prognostic prediction models mostly rely on clinicopathological features obtained from retrospective analysis [6,7]. However, studies have found that the prediction accuracy of these models is limited [8–10]. As a non-invasive method, a blood-based biomarker analysis is more attractive for various cancers [11,12]. At the same time, much evidence suggests that clinical factors alone are not sufficient to predict the survival rate of patients with UC, and the systemic inflammatory response and nutritional deficiency might play a vital role in the development and progression of cancer [13]. The modified

Glasgow Prognostic Score (mGPS) (Table 1) is a combination of C-reactive protein (CRP) and albumin, reflecting the inflammation and nutritional status of patients, and has an independent prognostic value for patients with various cancers, such as liver, lung, and colon cancer [14–16].

Table 1. The modified Glasgow Prognostic Scores.

mGPS	Points Allocated
CRP ≤ 10 mg/L and albumin ≥ 35 g/L	0
CRP > 10 mg/L	1
CRP > 10 mg/L and albumin < 35 g/L	2

mGPS = modified Glasgow Prognostic Score; CRP = C-reactive protein.

Many studies have shown that the mGPS has an important predictive value in the treatment of UC. However, due to differences in treatment methods and tumor staging, the results are inconsistent [17]. It is necessary to evaluate the prognostic value of the mGPS in patients with UC using a pooled analysis. Meta-analyses provide more reliable and accurate estimates of outcomes than individual studies. The aim of this study was to evaluate the relationship between pretreatment mGPS and the survival of patients with UC.

2. Materials and Methods

2.1. Protocol

This study followed the 2020 Preferred Reporting Items for Systematic Reviews and Meta-Analyses (PRISMA) guideline [18] and was registered in PROSPERO (CRD42022356946).

2.2. Literature Search Strategy

We searched the literature in Embase, PubMed, and the Web of Science from inception to August 2022. The following search terms were used for literature retrieval: (upper urinary tract urothelial carcinoma OR upper urinary tract carcinoma OR upper-tract urothelial carcinoma OR UTUC), (bladder cancer OR bladder neoplasms OR bladder tumor), and (Glasgow prognostic score OR GPS). To avoid missing literature, we searched for a list of references to relevant reviews and meta-analyses. Differences were resolved through discussion or by third-party ruling.

2.3. Inclusion/Exclusion Criteria

The inclusion criteria for eligible studies were as follows: (1) patients were diagnosed with UC by histopathology; (2) research aimed at studying the relationship between mGPS and survival results in patients with UC, such as overall survival (OS), progression-free survival (PFS), recurrence-free survival (RFS), and/or cancer-specific survival (CSS); (3) the hazard ratio (HR) and 95% confidence interval (95% CI) of survival results were reported; (4) studies published in English as full-text articles; (5) mGPS scores were computed before treatment. The exclusion criteria were as follows: (1) repetitive articles; (2) experimental or non-human studies; (3) studies focusing on the relationship between GPS and survival outcomes in patients with UC; (4) reviews, editorials, case reports, letters, comments, meta-analyses, and conference abstracts; and (5) incomplete or unavailable data.

2.4. Data Extraction and Quality Assessment

Two researchers (D.T. and J.L.) independently extracted data from the eligible studies, and any differences between the two investigators were resolved via discussions or by a third-party decision. The following data were extracted from each study: first author, study area, publication year, sample size, research design, tumor type, tumor stage, patient age, survival outcome parameters, treatment strategy, and average follow-up. All survival results were directly expressed as HR and the corresponding 95% CI. When the data in the study were analyzed in both univariate and multivariate analyses, multivariate analysis data were used. The Newcastle–Ottawa Scale (NOS) was used to assess the quality of the included studies [19]. In this meta-analysis, studies were considered to be of high quality when the score was ≥7. The risk of bias of included studies was assessed using the Quality In Prognosis Studies (QUIPS) tool [20].

2.5. Statistical Analysis

All statistical analyses were performed using STATA v.14 (StataCorp, College Station, TX, USA). Pooled HRs with corresponding 95% CIs were used to assess the association between the mGPS and survival results. Heterogeneity among studies was evaluated using Cochran's Q and Higgins I^2 tests. $I^2 > 50\%$ or $p < 0.10$ noted significant heterogeneity. This meta-analysis used the random-effects model for summary analysis. A subgroup analysis of the primary survival outcome, OS, was conducted to explore the potential sources of heterogeneity. A sensitivity analysis was also conducted to assess the impact of individual research data on survival outcomes. HRs and 95% CIs were used to assess the relationship between mGPS and survival outcomes in UC. We did not evaluate publication bias because fewer than 10 available studies were not convincing [21].

3. Results

3.1. Study Selection

A total of 311 papers were retrieved from Embase, PubMed, and Web of Science databases. According to the PRISMA guidelines, a flow chart of the literature selection process is shown in Figure 1. After excluding unqualified studies, 13 studies including 12,524 patients were included in this pooled analysis [17,22–33].

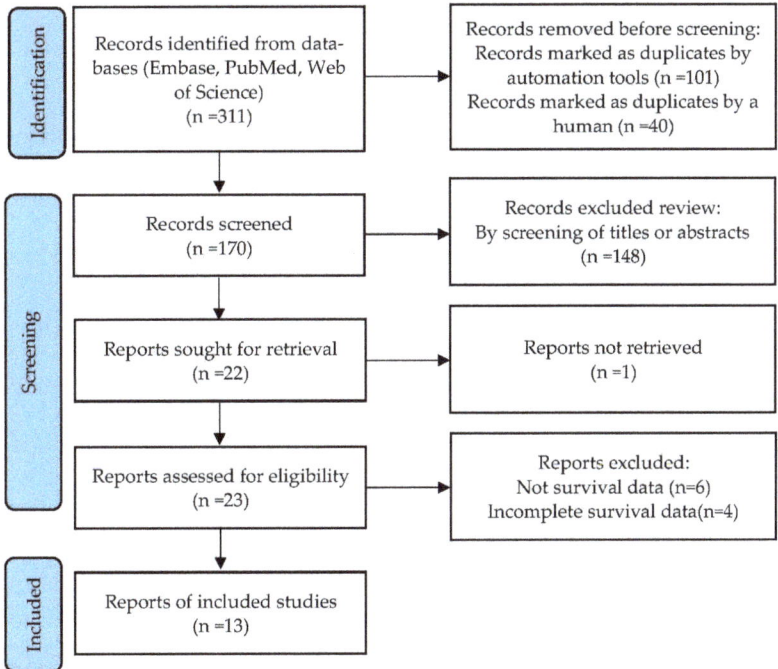

Figure 1. Flow diagram of literature search.

3.2. Study Characteristics

The main characteristics of the 13 included studies are presented in Table 2. All included studies were retrospective analyses and were published from 2013 to 2022. Seven studies were on BC [17,22–24,30,31,33], four studies were on UTUC [25–28], and two studies were on both BC and UTUC [29,32]. Six studies were conducted in Asia (China, Japan, and Korea) [23,25,26,28,30,32], and seven studies were conducted in Western countries (the United States, Italy, the United Kingdom, and Austria) [17,22,24,27,29,31,33]. The treatment methods include surgical treatment, immunotherapy, and chemotherapy. The sample size of the study ranged from 53 to 4335, and the median age of the patients ranged from 67 to 72 years. Eight studies reported a correlation between mGPS and OS [17,23,26–31], seven investigated the associations between mGPS and CSS [17,22,25,27,28,31,32], seven investigated the associations between mGPS and RFS [17,24,25,27,28,31,33], and five reported an association between mGPS and PFS [24,29,30,32,33]. Except for one study that only included evaluation data in the univariate analysis [30], most studies used multivariate analysis for evaluation. All studies had NOS scores > 7, except for Nagai [32], indicating that the overall quality of the included studies was high. The bias assessment is shown in Figure 2.

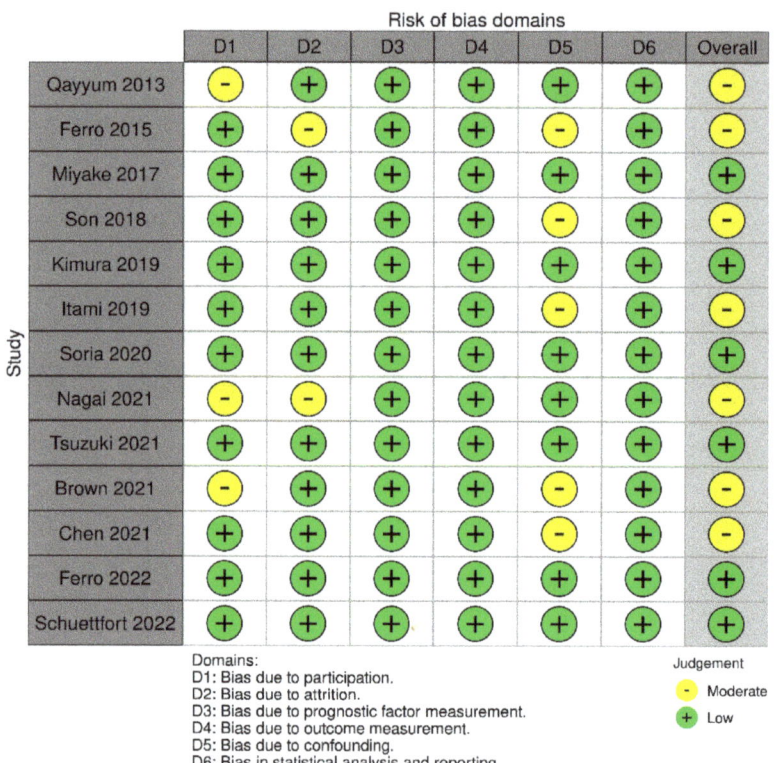

Figure 2. Risk of bias using the Quality in Prognosis Studies tool [20,34]. Low risk of bias; Moderate risk of bias [17,22–33].

3.3. mGPS and OS

Eight studies involving 8699 patients reported a correlation between mGPS and OS [17,23,26–31]. The summary analysis showed that there was a significant association between high pretreatment mGPS and worse survival rates (mGPS 1/0: HR = 1.33, 95% CI 1.12–1.58, p = 0.001; mGPS 2/0: HR = 2.02, 95% CI 1.43–2.84, p < 0.0001; mGPS high/low: HR = 2.48, 95% CI 1.48–4.14, p = 0.001) (Figure 3). At the same time, a subgroup analysis including the tumor type, treatment, ethnicity, and sample size was performed to explore possible sources of heterogeneity. The subgroup analysis showed similar results; high pre-treatment mGPS was significantly associated with poor OS (Table 3).

Table 2. Baseline characteristics of include studies and methodological assessment.

Author	Year	Country	Study Design	Tumor Type	mGPS Group	Treatment	Sample Size	Age (Years)	Analysis Method	Survival Analysis	Follow-Up (Months)	Quality Score
Qayyum et al. [22]	2013	United Kingdom	Retrospective	BC	High/low	Non-Surgery	68	Median72 (range, 43–93)	Multivariate	CSS	Median47 (range, 1.2–201)	8
Ferro et al. [17]	2015	Italy	Retrospective	BC	0/1/2	RC	1037	Median70 (range, 42–88)	Multivariate	RFS/OS/CSS	Median22 (range, 3–60)	9
Miyake et al. [23]	2017	Japan	Retrospective	BC	High/low	RC	117	Median72 (IQR, 61–77)	Multivariate	OS	Median22 (IQR, 10–64)	8
Son et al. [25]	2018	Korea	Retrospective	UTUC	0/1/2	RNU	1137	Median69 (IQR, 61–74)	Multivariate	RFS/CSS	Median39.1 (IQR, 18.3–63.8)	9
Kimura et al. [24]	2019	Austria	Retrospective	BC	0/1/2	TURB	1096	Median67 (IQR, 58–74)	Multivariate	PFS/RFS	Median64.8 (IQR, 26.5–110.9)	8
Itami et al. [26]	2019	Japan	Retrospective	UTUC	High/low	RNU	125	Median72 (range, 38–90)	Multivariate	OS	Median51 (range, 6–227)	8
Soria et al. [27]	2020	Italy	Retrospective	UTUC	0/1/2	RNU	2492	Median69 (IQR, 61–76)	Multivariate	RFS/CSS/OS	Median45 (IQR, 20–81)	9
Nagai et al. [32]	2021	Japan	Retrospective	mUC	High/low	shGC	68	-	Multivariate	CSS/PFS	-	6
Nagai et al. [32]	2021	Japan	Retrospective	mUC	High/low	PEM	74	-	Multivariate	CSS/PFS	-	6
Tsuzuki et al. [28]	2021	Japan	Retrospective	UTUC	0/1/2	RNU	273	Median71 (IQR, 63–77)	Multivariate	RFS/CSS/OS	Median36.1	8
Brown et al. [29]	2021	USA	Retrospective	mUC	0/1/2	ICIs	53	Median70 (range, 32–86)	Multivariate	PFS/OS	Median27.1	8
Chen et al. [30]	2021	China	Retrospective	BC	0/1/2	RC	267	-	Univariate	PFS/OS	-	8
Ferro et al. [33]	2022	Italy	Retrospective	BC	0/1/2	BCG	1382	Mean69.87 (IQR, 60.16–79.58)	Multivariate	PFS/RFS	Median44 (IQR, 36–58)	9
Schuettfort et al. [31]	2022	Austria	Retrospective	BC	0/1/2	RC	4335	Median67 (IQR, 60–73)	Multivariate	RFS/OS/CSS	Median41 (IQR, 18.3–60.8)	9

BC = bladder cancer; UTUC = upper urinary tract urothelial carcinoma; mGPS = modified Glasgow Prognostic Score; mUC = metastatic urothelial cell carcinoma; ICIs = immune checkpoint inhibitors; OS = overall survival; PFS = progression-free survival; RFS = recurrence-free survival; CSS = cancer-specific survival; RC = radical cystectomy; BCG = Bacillus Calmette-Guerin; TURB = transurethral resection of bladder; shGC = short hydration gemcitabine/cisplatin; PEM = pembrolizumab; RNU = remains radical nephroureterectomy; IQR = Interquartile Range.

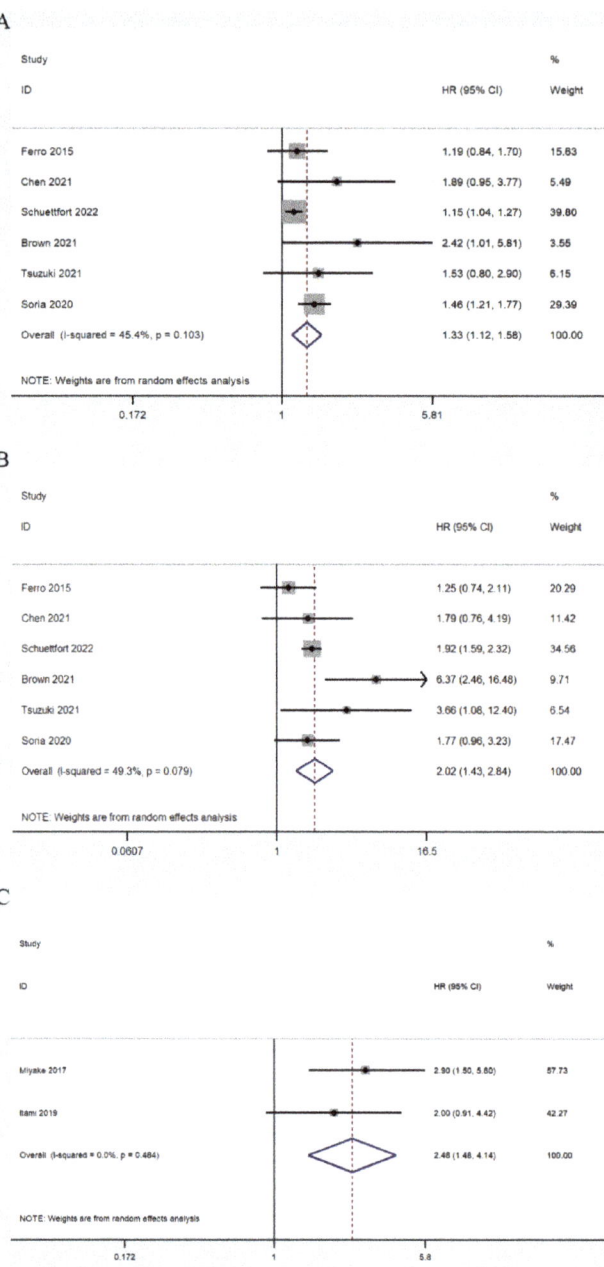

Figure 3. Forest plots of relationship between mGPS and OS in patients with urothelial carcinoma: (**A**) mGPS 1 vs. 0; (**B**) mGPS 2 vs. 0; (**C**) mGPS high vs. low [17,23,26–31].

Table 3. Subgroup analyses of OS.

Outcome	Variable	No. of Studies	Model	HR (95% CI)	p	Heterogeneity I^2 (%)	p
OS (1/0)	All	6	Random	1.33 (1.12, 1.58)	0.001	45.4	0.103
Ethnicity	Caucasian	4	Random	1.29 (1.07, 1.56)	0.008	58.0	0.068
	Asian	2	Random	1.69 (1.06, 2.70)	0.029	0.0	0.657
Tumor type	BC	3	Random	1.16 (1.06, 1.28)	0.002	0.0	0.368
	mUC	1	-	2.42 (1.01, 5.80)	0.048	-	-
	UTUC	2	Random	1.47 (1.22, 1.76)	0.000	0.0	0.891
Sample size	≤1500	4	Random	1.44 (1.09, 1.90)	0.009	3.8	0.374
	>1500	2	Random	1.28 (1.01, 1.61)	0.004	78.9	0.029
Treatment	Surgery	5	Random	1.29 (1.10, 1.51)	0.001	41.5	0.145
	Non-Surgery	1	-	2.42 (1.01, 5.80)	0.048	-	-
OS (2/0)	All	6	Random	2.02 (1.43, 2.84)	0.000	49.3	0.079
Ethnicity	Caucasian	4	Random	1.99 (1.29, 3.06)	0.002	65.6	0.033
	Asian	2	Random	2.26 (1.13, 4.54)	0.022	49.3	0.079
Tumor type	BC	3	Random	1.78 (1.42, 2.23)	0.000	12.4	0.319
	mUC	1	-	6.37 (2.46, 16.49)	0.000	-	-
	UTUC	2	Random	2.08 (1.15, 3.77)	0.015	8.4	0.296
Sample size	≤1500	4	Random	2.47 (1.15, 5.31)	0.020	69.3	0.021
	>1500	2	Random	1.91 (1.59, 2.28)	0.000	0.0	0.802
Treatment	Surgery	5	Random	1.85 (1.56, 2.18)	0.000	0.0	0.474
	Non-Surgery	1	-	6.37 (2.46, 16.49)	0.000	-	-

OS = overall survival; BC = bladder cancer; UTUC = upper urinary tract urothelial carcinoma; mUC = metastatic urothelial cell carcinoma; HR = hazard ratio; CI = confidence interval.

3.4. mGPS and PFS

Five studies involving 2940 patients reported the relationship between mGPS and PFS [24,29,30,32,33]. The summary analysis showed that high pretreatment mGPS in patients with UC was an independent predictor of PFS (mGPS 1/0: HR = 1.26, 95% CI 1.03–1.53, p = 0.021; mGPS 2/0: HR = 1.76, 95% CI 1.12–2.77, p = 0.013) (Figure 4).

3.5. mGPS and RFS

Seven studies involving 11,752 patients reported an association between mGPS and RFS [17,24,25,27,28,31,33]. The summary analysis showed that high pretreatment mGPS in patients with UC was an independent predictor of RFS (mGPS 1/0: HR = 1.36, 95% CI 1.18–1.56, p < 0.0001; mGPS 2/0: HR = 1.70, 95% CI 1.44–2.000, p < 0.0001) (Figure 5).

3.6. mGPS and CSS

Seven studies involving 9484 patients reported the relationship between mGPS and CSS [17,22,25,27,28,31,32]. The summary analysis showed that the association was not statistically significant between a score of 1 and poor CSS (mGPS 1/0: HR = 1.25, 95% CI 0.93–1.68, p = 0.133) (Figure 6A), but there was a significant association between high score and poor CSS before treatment (mGPS 2/0: HR = 1.81, 95% CI 1.30–2.52, p < 0.0001; mGPS high/low: HR = 2.31, 95% CI 1.58–3.37, p < 0.0001) (Figure 6B,C).

3.7. Sensitivity Analysis

A sensitivity analysis was conducted to assess the reliability of the merged OS, PFS, RFS, and CSS HRs (Figures S1–S4). The leave-one-out test showed that overall HR estimates of these survival results did not change significantly, indicating that the meta-analysis results were relatively stable and reliable.

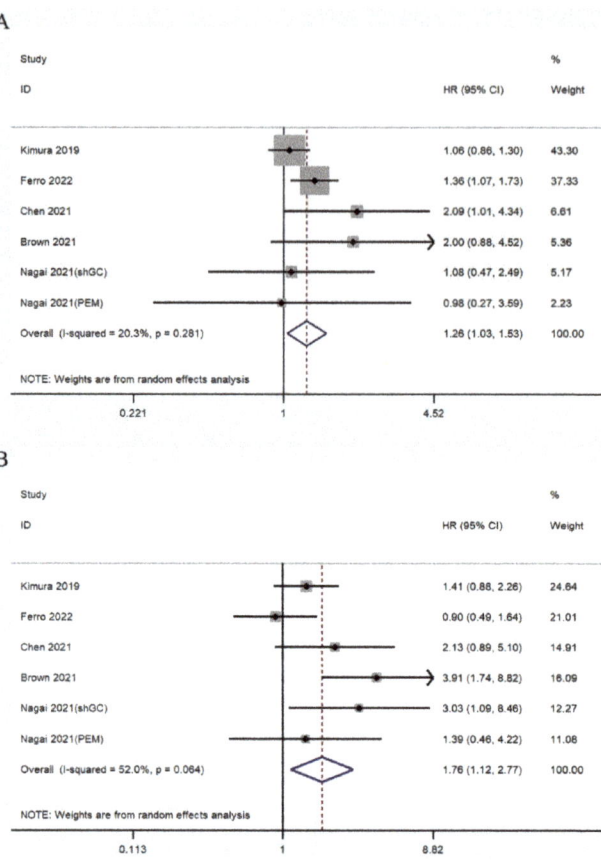

Figure 4. Forest plots of relationship between mGPS and PFS in patients with urothelial carcinoma: (**A**) mGPS 1 vs. 0; (**B**) mGPS 2 vs. 0 [24,29,30,32,33].

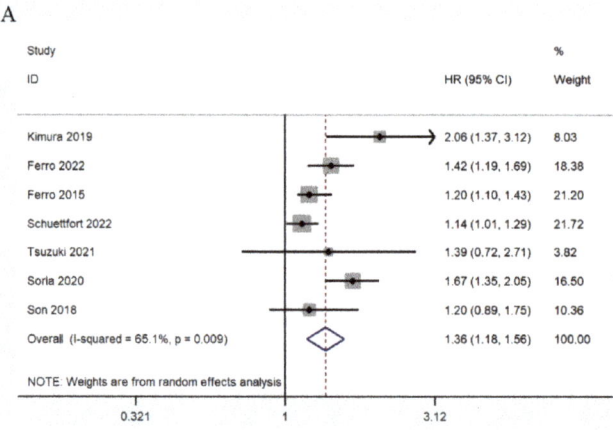

Figure 5. *Cont.*

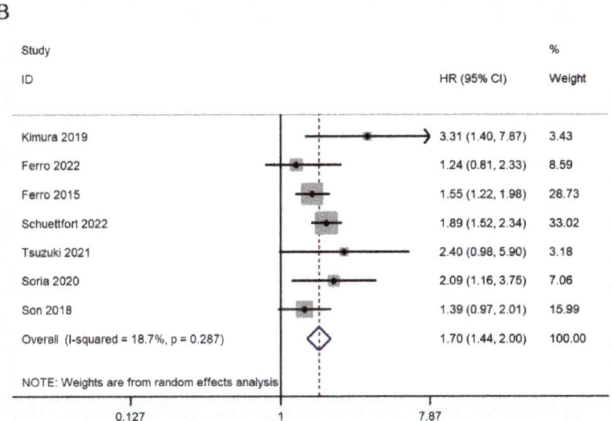

Figure 5. Forest plots of relationship between mGPS and RFS in patients with urothelial carcinoma: (**A**) mGPS 1 vs. 0; (**B**) mGPS 2 vs. 0 [17,24,25,27,28,31,33].

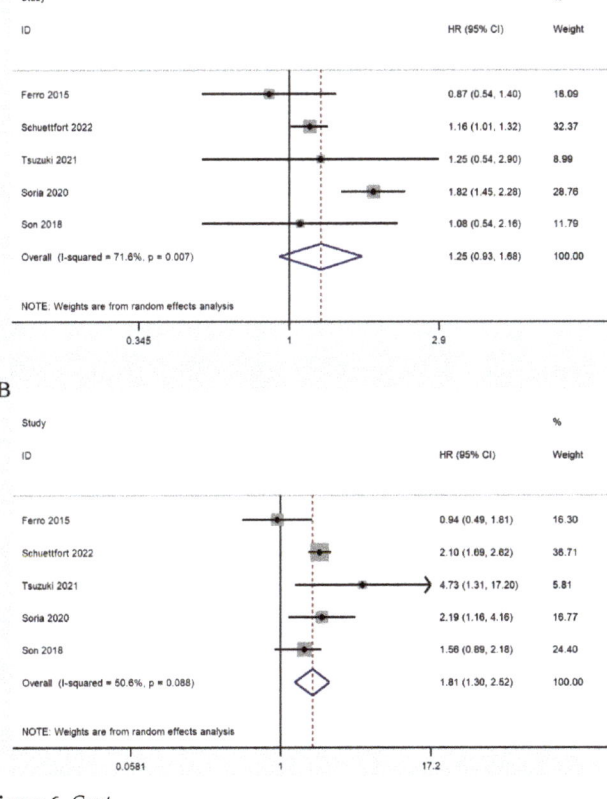

Figure 6. *Cont.*

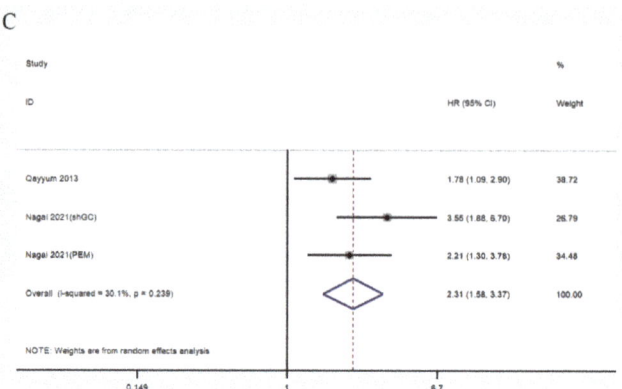

Figure 6. Forest plots of relationship between mGPS and CSS in patients with urothelial carcinoma: (**A**) mGPS 1 vs. 0; (**B**) mGPS 2 vs. 0; (**C**) mGPS high vs. low [17,22,25,27,28,31,32].

4. Discussion

This meta-analysis summarized all eligible studies, including 12,524 patients for the first time to evaluate the prognostic value of the mGPS in patients with UC. The results showed that a higher mGPS was closely related to lower survival (OS, PFS, RFS, and CSS). In view of the heterogeneity between studies, we conducted a subgroup analysis of OS based on the tumor type, treatment, ethnicity, and sample size. Our results show that the mGPS can be used as an independent predictor of the prognosis of UC.

The prognosis of patients with UC depends on the characteristics of the patient and the tumor. The transurethral resection of bladder tumors and postoperative adjuvant therapy are the main treatment methods for patients with non–muscle-invasive BC (NMIBC) [35]. In a postoperative study of Ta low-grade UC of the bladder, Mastroianni et al. found that gender and the European Organization for Research and Treatment of Cancer (EORTC) risk group are independent predictors of cancer recurrence, while the absence of the detrusor muscle does not affect RFS [36]. Cicione et al. showed that the ultrasound detection of the bladder detrusor wall's thickness increases the risk of recurrence and progression in patients with NMIBC [37]. Radical cystectomy is the standard treatment for localized muscle-invasive BC [38]. Even for elderly patients over 80 years old, the frailty index helps guide clinical decision making and, thus, improves patient prognosis [39,40]. Radical nephroureterectomy plus bladder cuff resection is the standard treatment for patients with high-risk non-metastatic UTUC [2]. To date, the most important histopathological prognostic variables are tumor stage and lymph node status after radical resections [38]. However, the surgical approach or completion with intracorporeal urinary diversion does not affect the survival of patients with UC [41,42].

Although clinical features such as tumor stage and lymph node status are the most important factors affecting prognosis, the prognosis of patients with similar clinical manifestations is different, which requires more controllable indicators to predict the prognosis of patients. Cancer-related inflammation is the seventh hallmark of cancer, and inflammatory cytokines produced by tumors and related host cells affect tumor characteristics, including survival, proliferation, angiogenesis, and the metastasis of malignant cells [43]. Therefore, in addition to individual patient and tumor characteristics, clinical markers such as the neutrophil-to-lymphocyte ratio, insulin-like growth factor-I and its binding protein, insulin-like growth factor-I binding protein-2 and -3, the platelet-lymphocyte ratio [44–46], molecular markers such as molecular subtypes, circulating tumor cells, and DNA damage repair-gene defects are also used to predict the prognosis of UC [47–49].

However, studies have shown that systemic inflammatory responses and nutritional deficiencies may play crucial roles in the development and progression of human cancer. CRP is a marker of systemic inflammation and has been used to determine the prognosis and predict the clinical results of cancer patients [50]. Serum albumin is one of the most common nutritional indicators and is often used to assess nutritional statuses, disease severity, disease progression, and prognosis [51]. Hypoproteinemia is often associated with nutritional deficiencies, poor working conditions, and weight loss, and it negatively impacts the prognosis of cancer patients [52]. The GPS, first described by Forrest et al. [53,54], combined serum albumin and CRP levels and could provide more comprehensive and accurate prognostic information than using albumin or CRP alone, and it could simultaneously assess the patient's inflammation and nutritional status. Further studies by McMillan et al. showed that the CSS of patients with simple hypoalbuminemia was significantly higher than that of patients with elevated CRP levels. Therefore, the GPS was modified, and only one point was assigned to an elevated CRP concentration [55]. Proctor also found that low albumin level was unrelated to the low survival rate of some cancers (gastroesophageal, bladder, prostate, gynecological, renal, colorectal, neck, hepatopancreaticobiliary, and head) in a larger cohort study, indicating that the mGPS had greater consistency and a better prognostic value than that of the GPS [56].

Ferro et al. study found that mGPS is associated with smoking habits, high tumor grade, and concomitant carcinoma in situ in UC [17]. Qayyum et al. also showed that high mGPS is directly related to tumor stage, grade, and progression in UC [22]. Several meta-analyses have also discussed the prognostic role of mGPS in solid tumors. Jiang summarized and analyzed the data of 72 studies and found that mGPS had a medium predictive ability for OS, DFS, and CSS in esophageal cancer [57]. Wu summarized 25 studies that found that an elevated mGPS before treatment was a sign of poor prognosis in patients with pancreatic cancer [58]. In addition, mGPS is obtained from blood samples, has low cost and high efficiency, is easy to obtain and promote, and can be obtained before treatment. Therefore, we searched the relevant literature and performed a meta-analysis. A summary analysis of 13 studies determined that the higher the mGPS score, the worse the survival results (OS, PFS, RFS, and CSS) of patients. We also confirmed that mGPS had a predictive effect on OS, PFS, RFS, and CSS in patients with UC. These analyses indicate that a high mGPS is closely related to low survival rate in patients with UC. Pre-treatment mGPS is a powerful prognostic marker for patients with UC, which helps guide clinical practice and make appropriate treatment decisions.

Although this analysis systematically analyzed the predictive value of the mGPS for patients with UC before treatment, there are still some limitations. All included studies were retrospective studies with increasing bias. The patients included in the study had substantial differences in pathological staging and treatment methods, which may have led to different survival results and increased heterogeneity among the studies. In addition, in the included studies, there is a great difference in postoperative adjuvant therapy, which is difficult to analyze. The reason is that the adjuvant therapy was mostly determined by the therapist according to guideline recommendations. Moreover, postoperative management strategies vary in different regions and centers, most of the research cycles were long, and the adjuvant therapy guidelines were constantly revised over time. To overcome these limitations, further multicenter prospective studies with larger sample sizes are needed.

5. Conclusions

This meta-analysis confirms the close relationship between a high mGPS and the poor prognosis of UC. The mGPS is a simple, effective, and practical prognostic biomarker that can provide an important reference for clinical decision making in the treatment of UC. However, large-scale prospective studies are required before widespread clinical applications.

Supplementary Materials: The following supporting information can be downloaded at: https://www.mdpi.com/article/10.3390/jcm11216261/s1, Figure S1. Sensitivity analysis of the effect of modified Glasgow prognostic score on overall survival in urothelial carcinoma: (A) mGPS 1 vs. 0; (B) mGPS 2 vs. 0; (C) mGPS high vs. low. Figure S2. Sensitivity analysis of the effect of modified Glasgow prognostic score on progression free survival in urothelial carcinoma: (A) mGPS 1 vs. 0; (B) mGPS 2 vs. 0. Figure S3. Sensitivity analysis of the effect of modified Glasgow prognostic score on recurrence free survival in urothelial carcinoma: (A) mGPS 1 vs. 0; (B) mGPS 2 vs. 0. Figure S4. Sensitivity analysis of the effect of modified Glasgow prognostic score on cancer specific survival in urothelial carcinoma: (A) mGPS 1 vs. 0; (B) mGPS 2 vs. 0; (C) mGPS high vs. low.

Author Contributions: Conceptualization, P.T., T.L., P.Z. and Q.W.; methodology, software, formal analysis, and data curation, D.T., J.Z., Q.X., J.J., Y.L. and J.L.; writing—original draft preparation, D.T.; writing—review and editing, D.T., J.L. and Q.W. All authors have read and agreed to the published version of the manuscript.

Funding: This research received no external funding.

Institutional Review Board Statement: Not applicable.

Informed Consent Statement: Not applicable.

Data Availability Statement: Not applicable.

Conflicts of Interest: The authors declare no conflict of interest.

References

1. Ahmadi, H.; Duddalwar, V.; Daneshmand, S. Diagnosis and Staging of Bladder Cancer. *Hematol Oncol Clin. N. Am* **2021**, *35*, 531–541.
2. Rouprêt, M.; Babjuk, M.; Burger, M.; Capoun, O.; Cohen, D.; Compérat, E.M.; Cowan, N.C.; Dominguez-Escrig, J.L.; Gontero, P.; Hugh Mostafid, A.; et al. European Association of Urology Guidelines on Upper Urinary Tract Urothelial Carcinoma: 2020 Update. *Eur. Urol.* **2021**, *79*, 62–79.
3. Terakawa, T.; Miyake, H.; Muramaki, M.; Takenaka, A.; Hara, I.; Fujisawa, M. Risk Factors for Intravesical Recurrence After Surgical Management of Transitional Cell Carcinoma of the Upper Urinary Tract. *Urology* **2008**, *71*, 123–127.
4. Katims, A.B.; Say, R.; Derweesh, I.; Uzzo, R.; Minervini, A.; Wu, Z.; Abdollah, F.; Sundaram, C.; Ferro, M.; Rha, K.; et al. Risk Factors for Intravesical Recurrence after Minimally Invasive Nephroureterectomy for Upper Tract Urothelial Cancer (ROBUUST Collaboration). *J. Urol.* **2021**, *206*, 568–576.
5. Elawdy, M.M.; Osman, Y.; Taha, D.E.; Zahran, M.H.; El-Halwagy, S.; Garba, M.E.; Harraz, A.M. Risk factors and prognosis of intravesical recurrence after surgical management of upper tract urothelial carcinoma: A 30-year single centre experience. *Arab. J. Urol.* **2019**, *15*, 216–222.
6. Fernandez-Gomez, J.; Madero, R.; Solsona, E.; Unda, M.; Martinez-Piñeiro, L.; Gonzalez, M.; Portillo, J.; Ojea, A.; Pertusa, C.; Rodriguez-Molina, J.; et al. Predicting nonmuscle invasive bladder cancer recurrence and progression in patients treated with bacillus Calmette-Guerin: The CUETO scoring model. *J. Urol.* **2009**, *182*, 2195–2203.
7. Sylvester, R.J.; van der Meijden, A.P.M.; Oosterlinck, W.; Witjes, J.A.; Bouffioux, C.; Denis, L.; Newling, D.W.W.; Kurth, K. Predicting Recurrence and Progression in Individual Patients with Stage Ta T1 Bladder Cancer Using EORTC Risk Tables: A Combined Analysis of 2596 Patients from Seven EORTC Trials. *Eur. Urol.* **2006**, *49*, 466–477.
8. Fernandez-Gomez, J.; Madero, R.; Solsona, E.; Unda, M.; Martinez-Piñeiro, L.; Ojea, A.; Portillo, J.; Montesinos, M.; Gonzalez, M.; Pertusa, C.; et al. The EORTC Tables Overestimate the Risk of Recurrence and Progression in Patients with Non–Muscle-Invasive Bladder Cancer Treated with Bacillus Calmette-Guérin: External Validation of the EORTC Risk Tables. *Eur. Urol.* **2011**, *60*, 423–430.
9. Xylinas, E.; Kent, M.; Kluth, L.; Pycha, A.; Comploj, E.; Svatek, R.S.; Lotan, Y.; Trinh, Q.D.; Karakiewicz, P.I.; Holmang, S.; et al. Accuracy of the EORTC risk tables and of the CUETO scoring model to predict outcomes in non-muscle-invasive urothelial carcinoma of the bladder. *Br. J. Cancer* **2013**, *109*, 1460–1466.
10. Chung, J.-W.; Kim, J.W.; Lee, E.H.; Chun, S.Y.; Park, D.J.; Byeon, K.H.; Choi, S.H.; Lee, J.N.; Kim, B.S.; Tae, H.; et al. Prognostic Significance of the Neutrophil-to-Lymphocyte Ratio in Patients with Non-Muscle Invasive Bladder Cancer treated with Intravesical Bacillus Calmette–Guérin and the Relationship with the CUETO Scoring Model. *Urol. J.* **2021**, *18*, 6765.
11. Hauth, F.; Roberts, H.J.; Hong, T.S.; Duda, D.G. Leveraging Blood-Based Diagnostics to Predict Tumor Biology and Extend the Application and Personalization of Radiotherapy in Liver Cancers. *Int. J. Mol. Sci.* **2022**, *23*, 1926.
12. Schuurbiers, M.; Huang, Z.; Saelee, S.; Javey, M.; de Visser, L.; van den Broek, D.; Monkhorst, K.; Heuvel Mvd Lovejoy, A.F.; Klass, D. Biological and technical factors in the assessment of blood-based tumor mutational burden (bTMB) in patients with NSCLC. *J. ImmunoTherapy Cancer* **2022**, *10*, e004064.
13. Grivennikov, S.I.; Greten, F.R.; Karin, M. Immunity, Inflammation, and Cancer. *Cell* **2010**, *140*, 883–899.

4. Ni, X.-C.; Yi, Y.; Fu, Y.-P.; He, H.-W.; Cai, X.-Y.; Wang, J.-X.; Zhou, J.; Cheng, Y.-F.; Jin, J.-J.; Fan, J.; et al. Prognostic Value of the Modified Glasgow Prognostic Score in Patients Undergoing Radical Surgery for Hepatocellular Carcinoma. *Medicine* **2015**, *94*, e1486.
5. Chen, Z.; Nonaka, H.; Onishi, H.; Nakatani, E.; Sato, Y.; Funayama, S.; Watanabe, H.; Komiyama, T.; Kuriyama, K.; Marino, K.; et al. Modified Glasgow Prognostic Score is predictive of prognosis for non-small cell lung cancer patients treated with stereotactic body radiation therapy: A retrospective study. *J. Radiat. Res.* **2021**, *62*, 457–464.
6. Golder, A.M.; McMillan, D.C.; Park, J.H.; Mansouri, D.; Horgan, P.G.; Roxburgh, C.S. The prognostic value of combined measures of the systemic inflammatory response in patients with colon cancer: An analysis of 1700 patients. *Br. J. Cancer* **2021**, *124*, 1828–1835.
7. Ferro, M.; De Cobelli, O.; Buonerba, C.; Di Lorenzo, G.; Capece, M.; Bruzzese, D.; Autorino, R.; Bottero, D.; Cioffi, A.; Matei, D.V.; et al. Modified Glasgow Prognostic Score is Associated with Risk of Recurrence in Bladder Cancer Patients After Radical Cystectomy. *Medicine* **2015**, *94*, e1861.
8. Page, M.J.; McKenzie, J.E.; Bossuyt, P.M.; Boutron, I.; Hoffmann, T.C.; Mulrow, C.D.; Shamseer, L.; Tetzlaff, J.M.; Akl, E.A.; Brennan, S.E.; et al. The PRISMA 2020 statement: An updated guideline for reporting systematic reviews. *BMJ* **2021**, *372*, n71.
9. Stang, A. Critical evaluation of the Newcastle-Ottawa scale for the assessment of the quality of nonrandomized studies in meta-analyses. *Eur. J. Epidemiol.* **2010**, *25*, 603–605.
10. Hayden, J.A.; van der Windt, D.A.; Cartwright, J.L.; Côté, P.; Bombardier, C. Assessing bias in studies of prognostic factors. *Ann. Intern. Med.* **2013**, *158*, 280–286.
11. Sternea, J.A.C.; Gavaghanb, D.; Egger, M. Publication and related bias in meta-analysis: Power of statistical tests and prevalence in the literature. *J. Clin. Epidemiol.* **2000**, *53*, 1119–1129.
12. Qayyum, T.; McArdle, P.; Hilmy, M.; Going, J.; Orange, C.; Seywright, M.; Horgan, P.; Underwood, M.; Edwards, J. A Prospective Study of the Role of Inflammation in Bladder Cancer. *Curr. Urol.* **2013**, *6*, 189–193.
13. Miyake, M.; Morizawa, Y.; Hori, S.; Marugami, N.; Iida, K.; Ohnishi, K.; Gotoh, D.; Tatsumi, Y.; Nakai, Y.; Inoue, T.; et al. Integrative Assessment of Pretreatment Inflammation-, Nutrition-, and Muscle-Based Prognostic Markers in Patients with Muscle-Invasive Bladder Cancer Undergoing Radical Cystectomy. *Oncology* **2017**, *93*, 259–269.
14. Kimura, S.; D' Andrea, D.; Soria, F.; Foerster, B.; Abufaraj, M.; Vartolomei, M.D.; Iwata, T.; Karakiewicz, P.I.; Rink, M.; Gust, K.M.; et al. Prognostic value of modified Glasgow Prognostic Score in non–muscle-invasive bladder cancer. *Urol. Oncol. Semin. Orig. Investig.* **2019**, *37*, e119–e179.
15. Son, S.; Hwang, E.-C.; Jung, S.-I.; Kwon, D.-D.; Choi, S.-H.; Kwon, T.-G.; Noh, J.-H.; Kim, M.-K.; Seo, I.-Y.; Kim, C.-S.; et al. Prognostic value of preoperative systemic inflammation markers in localized upper tract urothelial cell carcinoma: A large, multicenter cohort analysis. *Minerva Urol. Nephrol.* **2018**, *70*, 300–309.
16. Itami, Y.; Miyake, M.; Tatsumi, Y.; Gotoh, D.; Hori, S.; Morizawa, Y.; Iida, K.; Ohnishi, K.; Nakai, Y.; Inoue, T.; et al. Preoperative predictive factors focused on inflammation-, nutrition-, and muscle-status in patients with upper urinary tract urothelial carcinoma undergoing nephroureterectomy. *Int. J. Clin. Oncol.* **2019**, *24*, 533–545.
17. Soria, F.; Giordano, A.; D'Andrea, D.; Moschini, M.; Rouprêt, M.; Margulis, V.; Karakiewicz, P.I.; Briganti, A.; Bensalah, K.; Mathieu, R.; et al. Prognostic value of the systemic inflammation modified Glasgow prognostic score in patients with upper tract urothelial carcinoma (UTUC) treated with radical nephroureterectomy: Results from a large multicenter international collaboration. *Urol. Oncol. Semin. Orig. Investig.* **2020**, *38*, e602–e611.
18. Tsuzuki, S.; Kimura, S.; Fukuokaya, W.; Yanagisawa, T.; Hata, K.; Miki, J.; Kimura, T.; Abe, H.; Egawa, S. Modified Glasgow prognostic score is a pre-surgical prognostic marker of disease mortality in upper urinary tract urothelial carcinoma. *Jpn. J. Clin. Oncol.* **2021**, *51*, 138–144.
19. Brown, J.T.; Liu, Y.; Shabto, J.M.; Martini, D.J.; Ravindranathan, D.; Hitron, E.E.; Russler, G.A.; Caulfield, S.; Yantorni, L.B.; Joshi, S.S.; et al. Baseline Modified Glasgow Prognostic Score Associated with Survival in Metastatic Urothelial Carcinoma Treated with Immune Checkpoint Inhibitors. *Oncologist* **2021**, *26*, 397–405.
30. Chen, J.; Hao, L.; Zhang, S.; Zhang, Y.; Dong, B.; Zhang, Q.; Han, C. Preoperative Fibrinogen–Albumin Ratio, Potential Prognostic Factors for Bladder Cancer Patients Undergoing Radical Cystectomy: A Two-Center Study. *Cancer Manag. Res.* **2021**, *13*, 3181–3192.
31. Schuettfort, V.M.; Gust, K.; D'Andrea, D.; Quhal, F.; Mostafaei, H.; Laukhtina, E.; Mori, K.; Rink, M.; Abufaraj, M.; Karakiewicz, P.I.; et al. Impact of the preoperative modified Glasgow Prognostic Score on disease outcome after radical cystectomy for urothelial carcinoma of the bladder. *Minerva Urol. Nephrol.* **2022**, *74*, 302–312.
32. Nagai, T.; Naiki, T.; Isobe, T.; Sugiyama, Y.; Etani, T.; Iida, K.; Nozaki, S.; Noda, Y.; Shimizu, N.; Tasaki, Y.; et al. Modified Glasgow Prognostic Score 2 as a Prognostic Marker in Patients with Metastatic Urothelial Carcinoma. *Vivo* **2021**, *35*, 2793–2800.
33. Ferro, M.; Tătaru, O.S.; Musi, G.; Lucarelli, G.; Abu Farhan, A.R.; Cantiello, F.; Damiano, R.; Hurle, R.; Contieri, R.; Busetto, G.M.; et al. Modified Glasgow Prognostic Score as a Predictor of Recurrence in Patients with High Grade Non-Muscle Invasive Bladder Cancer Undergoing Intravesical Bacillus Calmette–Guerin Immunotherapy. *Diagnostics* **2022**, *12*, 586.
34. McGuinness, L.A.; Higgins, J.P.T. Risk-of-bias VISualization (robvis): An R package and Shiny web app for visualizing risk-of-bias assessments. *Res. Syn. Meth.* **2021**, *12*, 55–61.
35. Babjuk, M.; Burger, M.; Capoun, O.; Cohen, D.; Compérat, E.M.; Dominguez Escrig, J.L.; Gontero, P.; Liedberg, F.; Masson-Lecomte, A.; Mostafid, A.H.; et al. European Association of Urology Guidelines on Non–muscle-invasive Bladder Cancer (Ta, T1, and Carcinoma in Situ). *Eur. Urol.* **2022**, *81*, 75–94.

36. Mastroianni, R.; Brassetti, A.; Krajewski, W.; Zdrojowy, R.; Salhi, Y.A.; Anceschi, U.; Bove, A.M.; Carbone, A.; De Nunzio, C.; Fuschi, A.; et al. Assessing the Impact of the Absence of Detrusor Muscle in Ta Low-grade Urothelial Carcinoma of the Bladder on Recurrence-free Survival. *Eur. Urol. Focus* **2021**, *7*, 1324–1331.
37. Cicione, A.; Manno, S.; Ucciero, G.; Cantiello, F.; Damiano, R.; Lima, E.; Posti, A.; Balloni, F.; De Nunzio, C. A larger detrusor wall thickness increases the risk of non muscle invasive bladder cancer recurrence and progression: Result from a multicenter observational study. *Minerva Urol. E Nefrol. Ital. J. Urol. Nephrol.* **2018**, *70*, 310–318.
38. Witjes, J.A.; Bruins, H.M.; Cathomas, R.; Compérat, E.M.; Cowan, N.C.; Gakis, G.; Hernández, V.; Linares Espinós, E.; Lorch, A.; Neuzillet, Y.; et al. European Association of Urology Guidelines on Muscle-invasive and Metastatic Bladder Cancer: Summary of the 2020 Guidelines. *Eur. Urol.* **2021**, *79*, 82–104.
39. De Nunzio, C.; Cicione, A.; Leonardo, F.; Rondoni, M.; Franco, G.; Cantiani, A.; Tubaro, A.; Leonardo, C. Extraperitoneal radical cystectomy and ureterocutaneostomy in octogenarians. *Int. Urol. Nephrol.* **2010**, *43*, 663–667.
40. De Nunzio, C.; Cicione, A.; Izquierdo, L.; Lombardo, R.; Tema, G.; Lotrecchiano, G.; Minervini, A.; Simone, G.; Cindolo, L.; D'Orta, C.; et al. Multicenter Analysis of Postoperative Complications in Octogenarians After Radical Cystectomy and Ureterocutaneostomy: The Role of the Frailty Index. *Clin. Genitourin. Cancer* **2019**, *17*, 402–407.
41. Mastroianni, R.; Ferriero, M.; Tuderti, G.; Anceschi, U.; Bove, A.M.; Brassetti, A.; Misuraca, L.; Zampa, A.; Torregiani, G.; Ghiani, E.; et al. Open Radical Cystectomy versus Robot-Assisted Radical Cystectomy with Intracorporeal Urinary Diversion: Early Outcomes of a Single-Center Randomized Controlled Trial. *J. Urol.* **2022**, *207*, 982–992.
42. Mastroianni, R.; Tuderti, G.; Anceschi, U.; Bove, A.M.; Brassetti, A.; Ferriero, M.; Zampa, A.; Giannarelli, D.; Guaglianone, S.; Gallucci, M.; et al. Comparison of Patient-reported Health-related Quality of Life Between Open Radical Cystectomy and Robot-assisted Radical Cystectomy with Intracorporeal Urinary Diversion: Interim Analysis of a Randomised Controlled Trial. *Eur. Urol. Focus* **2022**, *8*, 465–471.
43. Colotta, F.; Allavena, P.; Sica, A.; Garlanda, C.; Mantovani, A. Cancer-related inflammation, the seventh hallmark of cancer: Links to genetic instability. *Carcinogenesis* **2009**, *30*, 1073–1081.
44. Miyama, Y.; Kaneko, G.; Nishimoto, K.; Yasuda, M. Lower neutrophil-to-lymphocyte ratio and positive programmed cell death ligand-1 expression are favorable prognostic markers in patients treated with pembrolizumab for urothelial carcinoma. *Cancer Med.* **2022**. [CrossRef]
45. Sari Motlagh, R.; Schuettfort, V.M.; Mori, K.; Katayama, S.; Rajwa, P.; Aydh, A.; Grossmann, N.C.; Laukhtina, E.; Pradere, B.; Mostafai, H.; et al. Prognostic impact of insulin-like growth factor-I and its binding proteins, insulin-like growth factor-I binding protein-2 and -3, on adverse histopathological features and survival outcomes after radical cystectomy. *Int. J. Urol.* **2022**, *29*, 676–683.
46. Jan, H.-C.; Hu, C.-Y.; Yang, W.-H.; Ou, C.-H. Combination of Platelet-Lymphocyte Ratio and Monocyte-Lymphocyte Ratio as a New Promising Prognostic Factor in Upper Tract Urothelial Carcinoma with Large Tumor Sizes > 3 cm. *Clin. Genitourin. Cancer* **2020**, *18*, e484–e500.
47. Sjödahl, G.; Abrahamsson, J.; Holmsten, K.; Bernardo, C.; Chebil, G.; Eriksson, P.; Johansson, I.; Kollberg, P.; Lindh, C.; Lövgren, K.; et al. Different Responses to Neoadjuvant Chemotherapy in Urothelial Carcinoma Molecular Subtypes. *Eur. Urol.* **2022**, *81*, 523–532.
48. Chiang, P.-J.; Xu, T.; Cha, T.-L.; Tsai, Y.-T.; Liu, S.-Y.; Wu, S.-T.; Meng, E.; Tsao, C.-W.; Kao, C.-C.; Chen, C.-L.; et al. Programmed Cell Death Ligand 1 Expression in Circulating Tumor Cells as a Predictor of Treatment Response in Patients with Urothelial Carcinoma. *Biology* **2021**, *10*, 674.
49. Vlachostergios, P.J. The interplay of cell cycle and DNA repair gene alterations in upper tract urothelial carcinoma: Predictive and prognostic implications. *Precis. Clin. Med.* **2020**, *3*, 153–160.
50. Wang, Y.; Wang, K.; Ni, J.; Zhang, H.; Yin, L.; Zhang, Y.; Shi, H.; Zhang, T.; Zhou, N.; Mao, W.; et al. Combination of C-Reactive Protein and Neutrophil-to-Lymphocyte Ratio as a Novel Prognostic Index in Patients with Bladder Cancer After Radical Cystectomy. *Front. Oncol.* **2021**, *11*, 762470.
51. Saito, H.; Kono, Y.; Murakami, Y.; Shishido, Y.; Kuroda, H.; Matsunaga, T.; Fukumoto Yo Osaki, T.; Ashida, K.; Fujiwara, Y. Postoperative Serum Albumin is a Potential Prognostic Factor for Older Patients with Gastric Cancer. *Yonago Acta Med.* **2018**, *61*, 72–78.
52. He, X.; Li, J.-P.; Liu, X.-H.; Zhang, J.-P.; Zeng, Q.-Y.; Chen, H.; Chen, S.-L. Prognostic value of C-reactive protein/albumin ratio in predicting overall survival of Chinese cervical cancer patients overall survival: Comparison among various inflammation based factors. *J. Cancer* **2018**, *9*, 1877–1884.
53. Forrest, L.M.; McMillan, D.C.; McArdle, C.S.; Angerson, W.J.; Dunlop, D.J. Evaluation of cumulative prognostic scores based on the systemic inflammatory response in patients with inoperable non-small-cell lung cancer. *Br. J. Cancer* **2003**, *89*, 1028–1030.
54. Forrest, L.M.; McMillan, D.C.; McArdle, C.S.; Angerson, W.J.; Dunlop, D.J. Comparison of an inflammation-based prognostic score (GPS) with performance status (ECOG) in patients receiving platinum-based chemotherapy for inoperable non-small-cell lung cancer. *Br. J. Cancer* **2004**, *90*, 1704–1706.
55. McMillan, D.C.; Crozier, J.E.M.; Canna, K.; Angerson, W.J.; McArdle, C.S. Evaluation of an inflammation-based prognostic score (GPS) in patients undergoing resection for colon and rectal cancer. *Int. J. Color. Dis.* **2007**, *22*, 881–886.

6. Proctor, M.J.; Talwar, D.; Balmar, S.M.; O'Reilly, D.S.J.; Foulis, A.K.; Horgan, P.G.; Morrison, D.S.; McMillan, D.C. The relationship between the presence and site of cancer, an inflammation-based prognostic score and biochemical parameters. Initial results of the Glasgow Inflammation Outcome Study. *Br. J. Cancer* **2010**, *103*, 870–876.
7. Jiang, Y.; Xu, D.; Song, H.; Qiu, B.; Tian, D.; Li, Z.; Ji, Y.; Wang, J. Inflammation and nutrition-based biomarkers in the prognosis of oesophageal cancer: A systematic review and meta-analysis. *BMJ Open* **2021**, *11*, e048324.
8. Wu, D.; Wang, X.; Sh, G.; Sun, H.; Ge, G. Prognostic and clinical significance of modified glasgow prognostic score in pancreatic cancer: A meta-analysis of 4629 patients. *Aging* **2021**, *13*, 1410–1421.

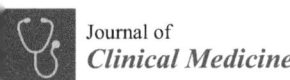

Article

Prognostic Significance of Organ-Specific Metastases in Patients with Metastatic Upper Tract Urothelial Carcinoma

Antonio Tufano [1,2,*], Nadia Cordua [2,3], Valerio Nardone [4], Raffaele Ranavolo [5], Rocco Simone Flammia [1], Federica D'Antonio [3], Federica Borea [3], Umberto Anceschi [6], Costantino Leonardo [1], Andrea Morrione [2] and Antonio Giordano [2,7,*]

1. Department of Urology, University Sapienza, 00185 Rome, Italy
2. Sbarro Institute for Cancer Research and Molecular Medicine, Center for Biotechnology, Department of Biology, College of Science and Technology, Temple University, Philadelphia, PA 19122, USA
3. Department of Biomedical Sciences, Humanitas University, 20072 Pieve Emanuele, Italy
4. Department of Precision Medicine, University of Campania "L. Vanvitelli", 80138 Naples, Italy
5. Urology Unit, AORN Ospedali dei Colli-Monaldi Hospital, 80131 Naples, Italy
6. Department of Urology, Regina Elena National Cancer Institute, 00144 Rome, Italy
7. Department of Medical Biotechnology, University of Siena, 53100 Siena, Italy
* Correspondence: antonio.tufano91@gmail.com (A.T.); president@shro.org (A.G.)

Abstract: Background: Existing data on metastatic upper tract urothelial carcinoma (mUTUC) are limited. In this study, we investigated the prognostic value of site-specific metastases in patients with mUTUC and its association with survival outcomes. Methods: We retrospectively collected data from the Surveillance, Epidemiology and End Results (SEER) database between 2004 and 2016. Kaplan–Meier analysis with a log-rank test was used for survival comparisons. Multivariate Cox regression was employed to predict overall survival (OS) and cancer-specific survival (CSS). Results: 633 patients were selected in this study cohort. The median follow-up was 6 months (IQR 2–13) and a total of 584 (92.3%) deaths were recorded. Within the population presenting with a single metastatic organ site, the most common metastatic sites were distant lymph nodes, accounting for 36%, followed by lung, bone and liver metastases, accounting for 26%, 22.8% and 16.2%, respectively. In patients with a single metastatic organ site, the Kaplan–Meier curves showed significantly worse OS for patients with liver metastases vs. patients presenting with metastases in a distant lymph node ($p < 0.001$), bone ($p = 0.023$) or lung ($p = 0.026$). When analyzing CSS, statistically significant differences were detectable only between patients presenting with liver metastases vs. distant lymph node metastases ($p < 0.001$). Multivariate analyses showed that the presence of liver (OS: HR = 1.732, 95% CI = 1.234–2.430, $p < 0.001$; CSS: HR = 1.531, 95% CI = 1.062–2.207, $p = 0.022$) or multiple metastatic organ sites (OS: HR = 1.425, 95% CI = 1.159–1.753, $p < 0.001$; CSS: HR = 1.417, 95% CI = 1.141–1.760, $p = 0.002$) was an independent predictor of poor survival. Additionally, survival benefits were found in patients undergoing radical nephroureterectomy (RNU) (OS: HR = 0.675, 95% CI = 0.514–0.886, $p = 0.005$; CSS: HR = 0.671, 95% CI = 0.505–0.891, $p = 0.006$) and chemotherapy (CHT) (OS: HR = 0.405, 95% CI = 0.313–0.523, $p < 0.001$; CSS: HR = 0.435, 95% CI = 0.333–0.570, $p < 0.001$). Conclusions: A distant lymph node was the most common site of single-organ metastases for mUTUC. Patients with liver metastases and patients with multiple organ metastases exhibited worse survival outcomes. Lastly, CHT administration and RNU were revealed to be predictors of better survival outcomes in the mUTUC cohort.

Keywords: metastatic upper tract urothelial carcinoma; metastatic organ; surveillance; Epidemiology and End Results; prognosis

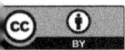

1. Introduction

Upper tract urothelial carcinoma (UTUC) is a rare malignancy that accounts for 5% to 10% of all urothelial cancers. The annual incidence of UTUC is typically estimated at 2 per 100,000 people in Western countries, with a peak in individuals aged from 70 to 90 years [1].

In patients with a diagnosis of UTUC, the 3-year overall survival (OS) rate is around 75% [2]. However, when considering metastatic UTUC (mUTUC) patients, the 3-year OS rate does not exceed 10% [3].

Recently, the prognostic role of metastasis at distant organs was investigated in multiple types of cancers [4–6]. To date, data on metastatic urothelium carcinoma are mainly based on studies on urothelial bladder cancer (UBC). For example, Shou et al. reported that the presence of liver metastasis was an independent predictor of OS when compared with other metastatic organ sites in metastatic bladder cancer (mBCa) [7]. Moreover, Dong et al. suggested that patients with mBCa exhibiting more than one metastatic site presented with unfavorable survival outcomes. Based on these results, we hypothesized that organ-specific metastases might also play a role in the prognosis of mUTUC [8].

Hence, our purpose was to retrospectively investigate the impact of organ-specific mUTUC patients on prognostic survival outcomes.

2. Materials and Methods

2.1. Database and Patient Selection

In January 2022, we interrogated the Surveillance, Epidemiology and End Results (SEER) database and identified patients with mUTUC from 2004 to 2016 according to the following inclusion criteria: (1) aged $\geq$ 18 years; (2) UTUC with distant metastasis as the first primary malignancy; (3) pathologically confirmed mUTUC of the renal pelvis, ureter or ureter orifice (International Classification of Disease for Oncology (ICD-O) site codes C65.9, C66.9 and C67.6, respectively); and (4) enrolled patients should have confirmed information on metastases in their bone, liver, lung, brain or distant lymph node. We excluded any metastatic pattern presented in less than 20 patients. The inclusion process is presented in Supplementary Figure S1. SEER*Stat software (SEER*Stat 8.2.3) was used to extract data.

2.2. Study Outcomes

Overall survival (OS) and cancer-specific survival (CSS) were the two major outcomes of this study. OS was defined as the interval of time from the UTUC diagnosis to death for any cause. CSS was defined as the interval from the date of UTUC diagnosis to death due to the tumor.

2.3. Statistical Analysis

Demographic factors were reported as frequency and proportion. The Mantel–Cox log-rank test was applied to compare the Kaplan–Meier survival curves for OS and CSS. Univariable and multivariable Cox proportional models with hazard ratios (HRs) and 95% confidence intervals (95% CIs) addressing both OS and CSS were performed. Two-sided p-values < 0.05 were considered significant. Statistical analysis was carried out using the Statistical Package for Social Sciences (SPSS) software v.26.0 (IBM Corp, Armonk, NY, USA).

3. Results

3.1. Demographic and Clinical Characteristics

The demographic characteristics of the included patients are shown in Table 1. A total of 633 mUTUC patients were identified after applying the inclusion/exclusion criteria. The median age at diagnosis was 72 years (IQR 63–79). mUTUC patients were more frequently males (57.8%) and ethnically white (83.6%). According to the AJCC Sixth edition TNM stage, 322 (50.9%) of the patients harbored a T-stage $\geq$ 2 and 431 (68.1%) had a positive N-stage. Furthermore, 354 (55.9%) mUTUC patients received chemotherapy (CHT) and 247

(39%) underwent radical nephroureterectomy (RNU). The median follow-up period was 6 months (IQR 2–13) and a total of 584 (92.3%) deaths were recorded.

Table 1. Baseline characteristics of patients with metastatic UTUC.

Characteristics	No.	%
Age (years)		
<65	176	27.8
≥65	457	72.2
Gender		
Female	267	42
Male	366	57.8
(T)NM		
X	151	23.8
0–2	160	25.3
3–4	322	50.9
T(N)M		
0	202	31.9
>1	431	68.1
Grade		
Low	159	25.1
High	474	74.9
Race		
White	529	83.6
Black	38	6.0
Other	66	10.4
Radiation		
No	54	8.5
Yes	122	19.3
Unknown	457	72.2
Radical nephroureterectomy		
No	386	61.0
Yes	247	39.0
Chemotherapy		
No	195	30.8
Yes	354	55.9
Unknown	84	13.3
Primary site		
Renal pelvis	427	67.5
Ureter	166	26.2
Ureteric orifice	40	6.3
Number of metastatic sites		
Single organ site	417	65.9
Multiple organ sites	216	34.1

3.2. Metastatic Patterns

Information on the metastatic organs is summarized in Table 1. Overall, 65.9% ($n = 417$) of the included population presented with a single metastatic organ site. Of those, the distribution showed that 36% ($n = 147$) were diagnosed with distant lymph nodes metastases, followed by lung, bone and liver metastases accounting for 26.0% ($n = 106$), 21.8% ($n = 89$) and 16.2% ($n = 66$), respectively. Moreover, 34.1% ($n = 216$) of patients presented with two or more metastatic organ sites.

3.3. Impact of Metastatic Sites and Treatment Scheme on Survival Outcomes

First, the OS and CSS were analyzed according to single- vs. multiple-organ metastases. Our results revealed that patients with a single metastatic organ site had significantly better outcomes for both OS ($p < 0.001$) and CSS ($p < 0.001$) (Figure 1a,b).

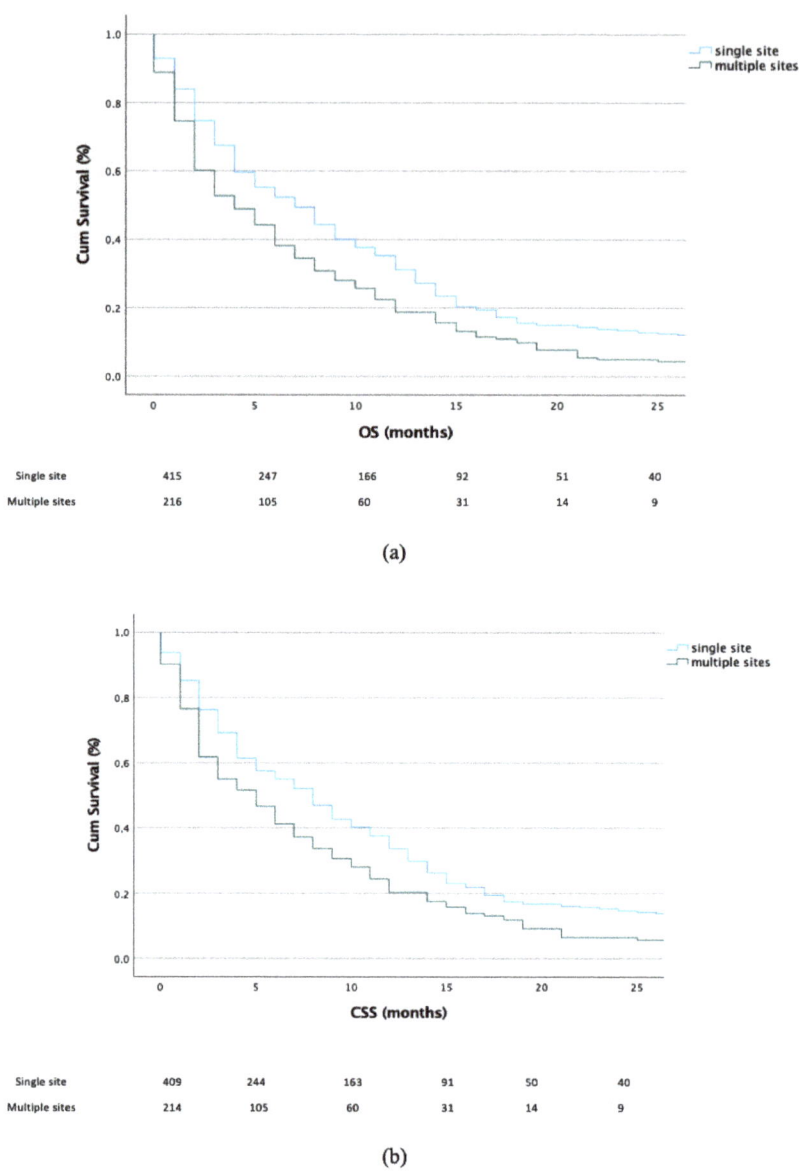

Figure 1. Kaplan–Meier plots depicting the OS (**a**) and CSS (**b**) according to single vs. multiple metastatic organ(s) patients.

Second, we focused on the OS and CSS in patients with a single metastatic organ site. Here, statistically significant differences were recorded between the Kaplan–Meier curves, showing worse outcomes in terms of OS for patients presenting liver metastases when compared with patients presenting distant lymph node ($p < 0.001$), bone ($p < 0.023$) and lung ($p < 0.026$) metastases (Figure 1a). Additionally, a difference was recorded between patients with lung vs. bone metastases ($p = 0.026$). When analyzing the CSS, a statistically significant difference was found only between liver vs. distant lymph node metastases ($p < 0.001$) (Figure 2a,b).

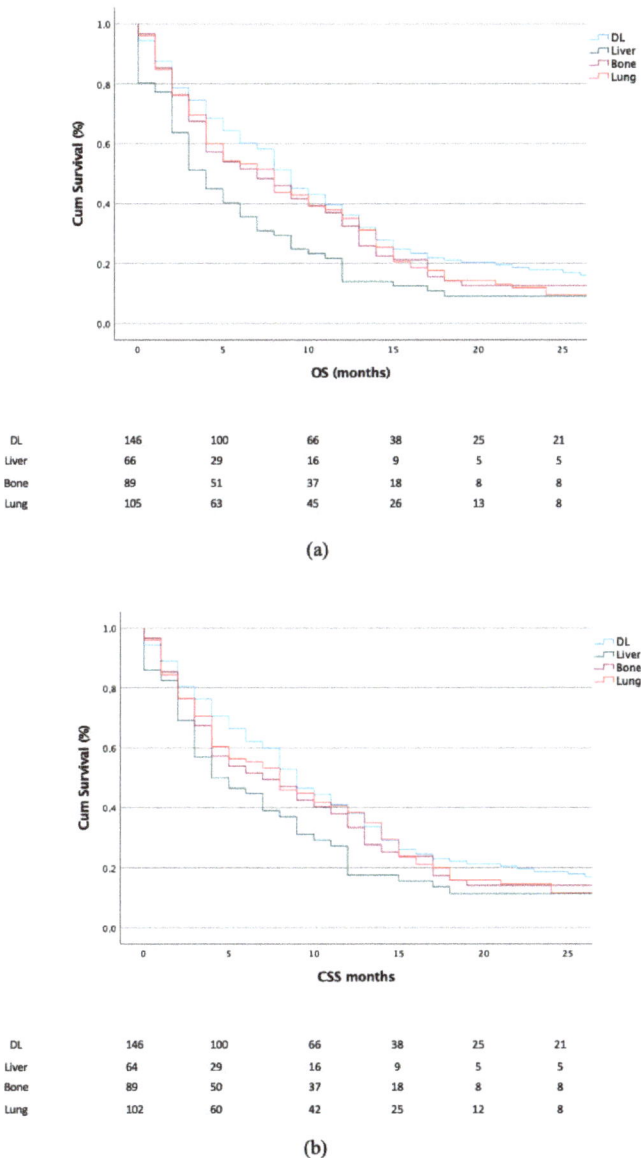

Figure 2. Kaplan–Meier plots depicting OS (**a**) and CSS (**b**) according to different metastatic organs in patients presenting single-organ metastases. DL, distant lymph node.

Third, we analyzed survival outcomes stratified by the treatment scheme (yes-CHT vs. no-CHT groups and yes-RNU vs. no-RNU groups) in patients harboring either single- or multiple metastatic organ sites.

Here, statistically significant differences were recorded, showing better survival outcomes in the yes-CHT vs. no-CHT group for both single- and multiple metastatic organ sites (OS and CSS: each $p < 0.001$). Additionally, in the subset of yes-CHT patients, better outcomes were recorded for single vs. multiple metastatic organ sites (OS: $p = 0.003$, CSS $p = 0.011$) (Figure 3a,b).

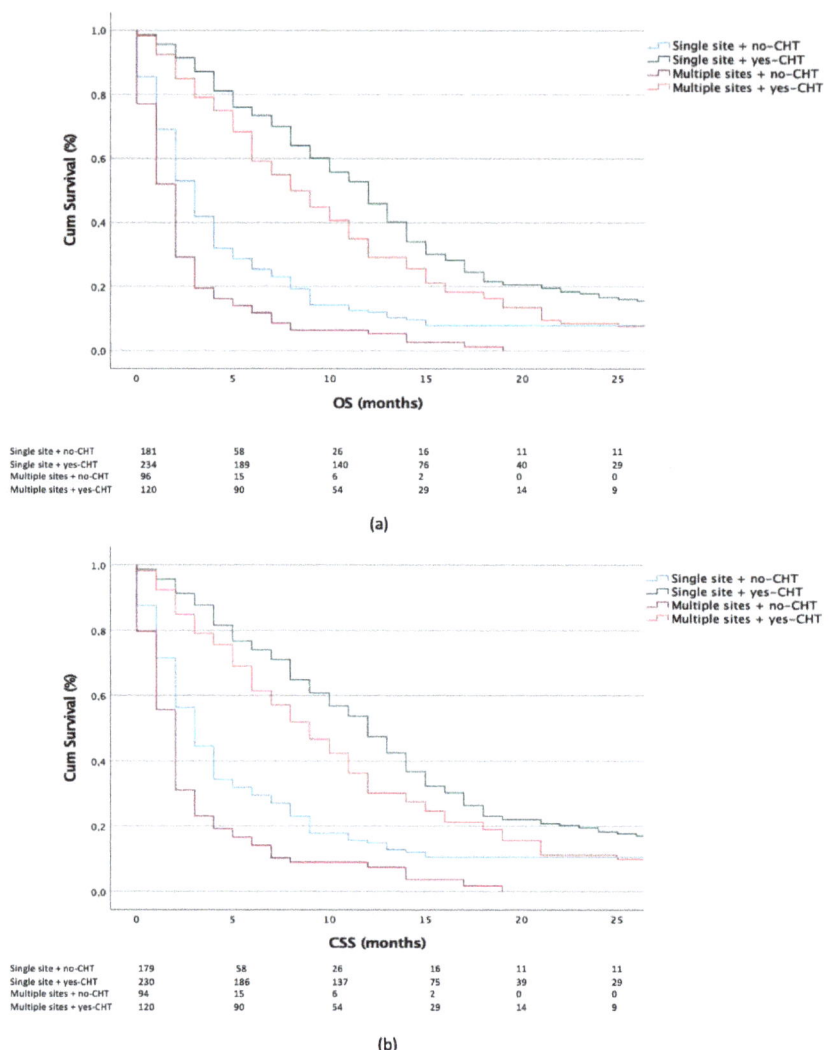

Figure 3. Kaplan–Meier plots depicting OS (**a**) and CSS (**b**) according to chemotherapy (CHT) administration in patients with single- vs. multiple-organ metastases.

When focusing on RNU treatment, we observed better survival outcomes in the yes-RNU vs. no-RNU group for single (OS: $p = 0.022$, CSS: $p = 0.010$) and multiple metastatic organ sites (OS and CSS: each $p < 0.001$). Lastly, in the subset of yes-RNU patients, better outcomes were observed in the single- vs. multiple-site groups (OS: $p = 0.197$, CSS $p = 0.234$) (Figure 4a,b).

The parameters age, sex, T-stage, N-stage, surgery of primary site, CHT and number of organ metastases were included in the multivariable Cox regression model (Table 2). Our analysis showed that the subgroup of patients presenting liver metastases had lower OS than patients with distant lymph node metastases (HR = 1.732, 95% CI: 1.234–2.430, $p < 0.001$). Similar results were found for CSS (HR = 1.531, 95% CI: 1.062–2.207, $p = 0.022$). Moreover, when comparing the number of metastatic organ sites (single vs. multiple), significantly longer OS (HR = 1.425, 95% CI: 1.159–1.753, $p = < 0.001$) and CSS (HR = 1.417, 95% CI: 1.141–1.760, $p = 0.002$) were observed in patients with single-organ metastases. Finally, patients undergoing RNU and CHT showed benefit in terms of OS and CSS (RNU—OS: HR = 0.675, 95% CI: 0.514–0.886, p = 0.005; CSS: HR = 0.671, 95% CI: 0.505–0.891; p = 0.006) (CHT—OS: HR = 0.405, 95% CI: 0.313–0.523, p < 0.001; CSS: HR = 0.435, 95% CI: 0.333–0.570, p < 0.001).

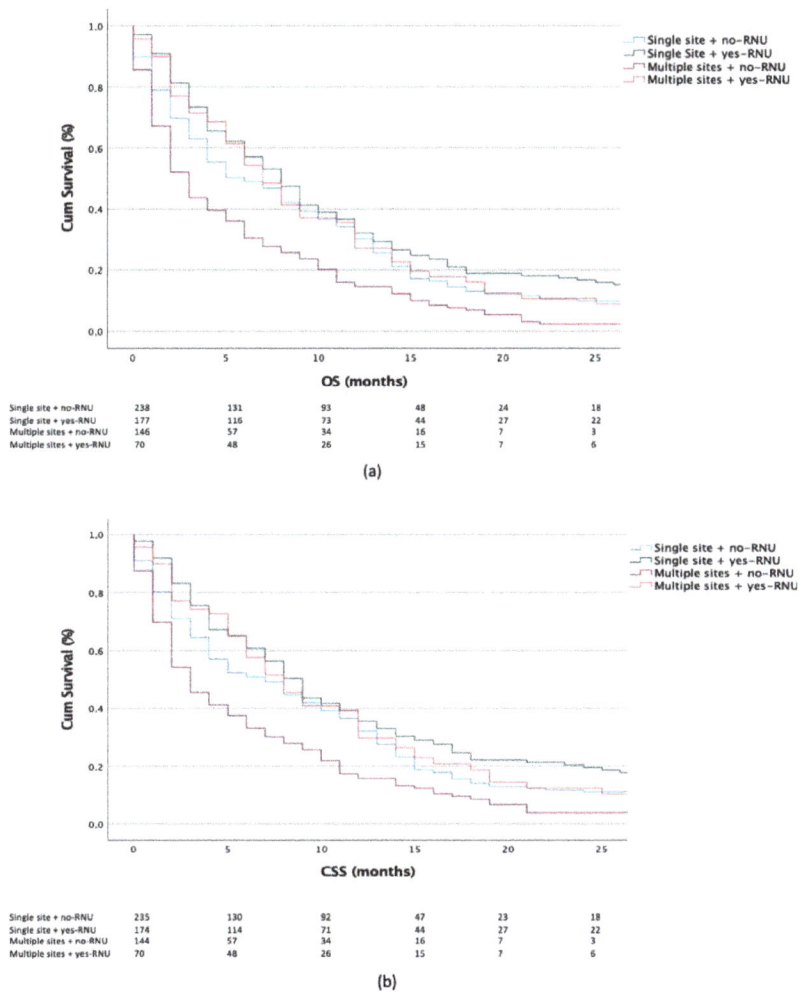

Figure 4. Kaplan–Meier plots depicting OS (**a**) and CSS (**b**) according to radical nephroureterectomy (RNU) treatment in patients with single- vs. multiple-organ metastases.

Table 2. Multivariate Cox regression analysis of factors that influenced OS and CSS outcomes.

Factors	Median OS (Months) HR (95% CI)	p-Value	Median CSS (Months) HR (95% CI)	p-Value
Age (years)				
<65	Reference			
≥65	1.196 (0.903–1.584)	0.213	1.167 (0.871–1.564)	0.301
Gender				
Female	Reference			
Male	0.900 (0.705–1.148)	0.394	0.946 (0.732–1.221)	0.946

Table 2. Cont.

Factors	Median OS (Months) HR (95% CI)	p-Value	Median CSS (Months) HR (95% CI)	p-Value
Tumor location				
Renal pelvis	Reference			
Ureter	0.782 (0.592–1.034)	0.085	0.715 (0.530–0.965)	0.028
Ureter orifice	1.044 (0.656–1.662)	0.855	1.023 (0.630–1.662)	0.926
(T)NM				
1–2	Reference			
3–4	1.16 (0.869–1.553)	0.312	0.946 (0.732–1.221)	0.668
T(N)M				
0	Reference			
≥1	0.962 (0.733–1.262)	0.777	1.003 (0.753–1.337)	0.983
Number of organ metastasis				
Single organ site	Reference			
Multiple organ sites	1.425 (1.159–1.753)	<0.001	1.417 (1.141–1.760)	0.002
Radical nephroureterectomy				
No	Reference			
Yes	0.675 (0.514–0.886)	0.005	0.671 (0.505–0.891)	0.006
Distant metastasis				
Lymph node	Reference			
Liver	1.732 (1.234–2.430)	0.001	1.531 (1.062–2.207)	0.022
Bone	1.188 (0.849–1.663)	0.315	1.219 (0.863–1.721)	0.261
Lung	1.179 (0.861–1.615)	0.304	1.138 (0.817–1.585)	0.444
Chemotherapy				
No	Reference			
Yes	0.405 (0.313–0.523)	<0.001	0.435 (0.333–0.570)	<0.001

4. Discussion

Previous studies demonstrated that advanced UTUC is aggressive and associated with a poor prognosis. At the time of diagnosis, 50–60% of patients with UTUC present locally advanced disease and up to 25% present with distant metastasis with a median OS of approximately 9 months [9–11]. These poor survival outcomes point out the fact that improving the treatment for this disease is still an essential issue and highlight the necessity to identify clinical factors that might improve clinical decision-making. Thus, in this study, we aimed at describing the pattern and frequency of metastatic sites and the prognostic relevance of any specific metastatic site by retrospectively analyzing a large patient cohort using the SEER database.

First, we observed important differences in metastatic sites, where we discovered a high frequency of distant lymph node metastases in patients that presented with a single metastatic organ site. These results are in disagreement with data reported from other mUTUC cohorts, as Chen et al. found that the lung represented the most common metastatic site, accounting for 42.3% of the whole cohort [12]. A possible interpretation of this difference might be that their analysis was limited to mUTUC presenting with a renal pelvis primary.

Second, our analysis focused on OS and CSS. Here, patients presenting with multiple metastases had worse OS and CSS according to Kaplan–Meier curves, which was confirmed using Cox regression analysis (OS: HR = 1.425, CSS: HR = 1.417). This finding is likely supported by the fact that the increase in tumor burden is usually associated with aggressive tumors and, at the same time, limits the possibility of a radical approach that can be used in oligometastatic patients (i.e., surgery or radiotherapy) [13]. Similar to our work, Li et al. analyzed the prognostic factors for OS in patients with mUTUC; the results of their multivariate analysis showed that the number of metastatic organs (1–2 vs. ≥3) outperformed the presence of visceral metastasis [14]. Additionally, Chen et al. reported that patients with ≤2 metastatic sites presented improved survival outcomes when compared with ≥3 metastatic sites [12].

Third, patients presenting with liver metastases had worse OS and CSS, as shown by the Kaplan–Meier curves. Our observations were also confirmed after multivariate adjustments for patient and tumor characteristics, where we identified a statistically significant OS and CSS disadvantage in patients with liver metastases relative to distant lymph node metastases (OS: HR = 1.732, CSS: HR = 1.531). Similarly, Dong et al. demonstrated that patients with liver metastases had worse OS rather than CSS, which provides a possible explanation [8]. Nonetheless, Shou et al. reported that mBCa patients with liver metastasis (SEER database; 2010–2014) exhibited worse OS compared with three other single metastatic organ sites [7]. A possible explanation for these results might be attributed to liver failure and, consequently, an increased overall mortality rate.

Fourth, our analyses focused on CHT administration. CHT is currently the accepted treatment option for advanced UTUC but the majority of data are extrapolated from UBC. In our cohort, CHT was associated with favorable OS (HR = 0.405) and CSS (HR = 0.435). Similar results were reported by Nazzani et al. in a non-surgically treated mUTUC population [15]. In our study, we confirmed the prognostic benefit of CHT in patients with either single or multiple metastatic organ sites. In contrast, Vassilakopoulou et al. demonstrated that adjuvant postoperative CHT does not add any significant benefit with regard to OS in high-risk UTUC patients [16]. However, in this cohort, patients with both locally advanced M0 and M+ were included. Unfortunately, within the SEER database, the proportion of patients that received cisplatin-based CHT vs. carboplatin-based CHT, as well as patients that received adjuvant vs. neoadjuvant CHT, is not specified. Moreover, we were unable to determine the rationale for determining patient exclusion from CHT regimens. However, we registered an administration rate of 55.9%, which is in line with the rates published by Browne et al. based on a large National Cancer Database (NCDB, 2004–2013) [17].

Sixth, we observed a statically significant association between radical nephroureterectomy (RNU) and OS (HR = 0.675) and CSS (HR = 0.671) after multivariable adjustments. Our findings are in agreement with several observational studies that addressed the role of surgery on primary tumor sites for mUTUC, especially in patients fit enough to receive cisplatin-based CHT [18,19].

Taken together, these data described the metastatic patterns of mUTUC and prognosis outcomes. Our results suggested that patients that presented with liver metastases had worse survival outcomes when compared with other metastatic sites. Moreover, patients that presented with metastasis at multiple secondary sites showed a worse prognosis, which was probably related to the greater burden of the disease. Nonetheless, CHT and RNU were found to be protective variables in the multivariate regression survival analysis.

We are aware of the limitations of our work, which should be interpreted in the context of its retrospective and population-based design. The SEER database included only five specific metastatic organs and the information reporting the number of metastases in each organ was not available. In addition, the SEER database does not ascertain either the type or delivery timing of chemotherapy. However, our analysis included a big population of mUTUC and our results can help to better understand and stratify prognoses, as well as justify more aggressive treatment strategies in oligometastatic patients.

5. Conclusions

Our analysis showed that a distant lymph node was the most common site of single-organ metastases for mUTUC. Patients with liver metastases and patients with multiple metastatic organ sites exhibited worse survival outcomes. Moreover, CHT administration and RNU were revealed to be predictors of better survival outcomes in the mUTUC cohort. These findings can be useful to stratify prognoses of mUTUC and justify aggressive treatment in oligometastatic patients.

Supplementary Materials: The following supporting information can be downloaded at: https://www.mdpi.com/article/10.3390/jcm11185310/s1, Figure S1: Flowchart of patients included.

Author Contributions: Conceptualization, A.T. and N.C.; methodology, A.M.; software, F.D.; validation, R.S.F. and A.M.; formal analysis, A.T. and V.N.; investigation, A.T. and N.C.; resources, A.G.; data curation, R.R. and F.B.; writing—original draft preparation, A.T. and N.C.; writing—review and editing, A.T. and A.M.; visualization, C.L.; supervision, A.G., A.M. and U.A.; project administration, A.T. and A.M.; funding acquisition, A.G. All authors have read and agreed to the published version of the manuscript.

Funding: The APC was funded by the Sbarro Health Research Organization.

Institutional Review Board Statement: Ethical review and approval were waived for this study due to the data being extracted from the SEER database.

Informed Consent Statement: Patient consent was waived due to the data being extracted from the SEER database.

Data Availability Statement: https://seer.cancer.gov, accessed on 1 July 2022.

Conflicts of Interest: The authors declare no conflict of interest.

References

1. Siegel, R.L.; Miller, K.D.; Fuchs, H.E.; Jemal, A. Cancer statistics, 2022. *CA Cancer J Clin.* **2022**, *72*, 7–33. [CrossRef] [PubMed]
2. Wang, Q.; Zhang, T.; Wu, J.; Wen, J.; Tao, D.; Wan, T.; Zhu, W. Prognosis and risk factors of patients with upper urinary tract urothelial carcinoma and postoperative recurrence of bladder cancer in central China. *BMC Urol.* **2019**, *19*, 24. [CrossRef] [PubMed]
3. Raman, J.D.; Messer, J.; Sielatycki, J.A.; Hollenbeak, C.S. Incidence and survival of patients with carcinoma of the ureter and renal pelvis in the USA, 1973–2005. *Br. J. Urol. Int.* **2011**, *107*, 1059–1064. [CrossRef] [PubMed]
4. Oweira, H.; Petrausch, U.; Helbling, D.; Schmidt, J.; Mannhart, M.; Mehrabi, A.; Schöb, O.; Giryes, A.; Decker, M.; Abdel-Rahman, O. Prognostic value of site-specific metastases in pancreatic adenocarcinoma: A Surveillance Epidemiology and End Results database analysis. *World J. Gastroenterol.* **2017**, *23*, 1872–1880. [CrossRef] [PubMed]
5. Wu, S.-G.; Li, H.; Tang, L.-Y.; Sun, J.-Y.; Zhang, W.-W.; Li, F.-Y.; Chen, Y.-X.; He, Z.-Y. The effect of distant metastases sites on survival in de novo stage-IV breast cancer: A SEER database analysis. *Tumour Biol. J. Int. Soc. Oncodevelopmental. Biol. Med.* **2017**, *39*, 1010428317705082. [CrossRef] [PubMed]
6. Abdel-Rahman, O. Clinical correlates and prognostic value of different metastatic sites in metastatic renal cell carcinoma. *Future Oncol.* **2017**, *13*, 1967–1980. [CrossRef] [PubMed]
7. Shou, J.; Zhang, Q.; Zhang, D. The prognostic effect of metastasis patterns on overall survival in patients with distant metastatic bladder cancer: A SEER population-based analysis. *World J. Urol.* **2021**, *39*, 4151–4158. [CrossRef] [PubMed]
8. Dong, F.; Fu, H.; Shi, X.; Shen, Y.; Xu, T.; Gao, F.; Wang, X.; Zhong, S.; Ding, Q.; Shen, Z.; et al. How do organ-specific metastases affect prognosis and surgical treatment for patients with metastatic upper tract urothelial carcinoma: First evidence from population based data. *Clin. Exp. Metastasis* **2017**, *34*, 467–477. [CrossRef] [PubMed]
9. Bellmunt, J.; von der Maase, H.; Mead, G.M.; Skoneczna, I.; De Santis, M.; Daugaard, G.; Boehle, A.; Chevreau, C.; Paz-Ares, L.; Laufman, L.R.; et al. Randomized phase III study comparing paclitaxel/cisplatin/gemcitabine and gemcitabine/cisplatin in patients with locally advanced or metastatic urothelial cancer without prior systemic therapy: EORTC Intergroup Study 30987. *J. Clin. Oncol. Off. J. Am. Soc. Clin. Oncol.* **2012**, *30*, 1107–1113. [CrossRef] [PubMed]
10. Rink, M.; Ehdaie, B.; Cha, E.K.; Green, D.A.; Karakiewicz, P.I.; Babjuk, M.; Margulis, V.; Raman, J.D.; Svatek, R.S.; Fajkovic, H.; et al. Stage-specific impact of tumor location on oncologic outcomes in patients with upper and lower tract urothelial carcinoma following radical surgery. *Eur. Urol.* **2012**, *62*, 677–684. [CrossRef] [PubMed]
11. Margulis, V.; Shariat, S.F.; Matin, S.F.; Kamat, A.M.; Zigeuner, R.; Kikuchi, E.; Lotan, Y.; Weizer, A.; Raman, J.; Wood, C.G.; et al. Outcomes of radical nephroureterectomy: A series from the Upper Tract Urothelial Carcinoma Collaboration. *Cancer* **2009**, *115*, 1224–1233. [CrossRef] [PubMed]
12. Chen, W.-K.; Wu, Z.-G.; Xiao, Y.-B.; Wang, Q.-Q.; Yu, D.-D.; Cai, J.; Zhou, C.-F. Prognostic Value of Site-Specific Metastases and Therapeutic Roles of Surgery and Chemotherapy for Patients with Metastatic Renal Pelvis Cancer: A SEER Based Study. *Technol. Cancer Res. Treat.* **2021**, *20*, 15330338211004914. [CrossRef] [PubMed]
13. Palma, D.A.; Olson, R.; Harrow, S.; Gaede, S.; Louie, A.V.; Haasbeek, C.; Mulroy, L.; Lock, M.; Rodrigues, G.B.; Yaremko, B.P.; et al. Stereotactic Ablative Radiotherapy for the Comprehensive Treatment of Oligometastatic Cancers: Long-Term Results of the SABR-COMET Phase II Randomized Trial. *J. Clin. Oncol. Off. J. Am. Soc. Clin. Oncol.* **2020**, *38*, 2830–2838. [CrossRef] [PubMed]
14. Li, X.; Li, S.; Chi, Z.; Cui, C.; Si, L.; Yan, X.; Mao, L.; Lian, B.; Tang, B.; Wang, X.; et al. Clinicopathological characteristics, prognosis, and chemosensitivity in patients with metastatic upper tract urothelial carcinoma. *Urol. Oncol.* **2021**, *39*, e1–e75. [CrossRef] [PubMed]
15. Nazzani, S.; Preisser, F.; Mazzone, E.; Marchioni, M.; Bandini, M.; Tian, Z.; Mistretta, F.A.; Shariat, S.F.; Soulières, D.; Montanari, E.; et al. Survival Effect of Chemotherapy in Metastatic Upper Urinary Tract Urothelial Carcinoma. *Clin. Genitourin. Cancer* **2019**, *17*, e97–e103. [CrossRef] [PubMed]

6. Vassilakopoulou, M.; Rouge, T.D.L.M.; Colin, P.; Ouzzane, A.; Khayat, D.; Dimopoulos, M.; Papadimitriou, C.A.; Bamias, A.; Pignot, G.; Nouhaud, F.X.; et al. Outcomes after adjuvant chemotherapy in the treatment of high-risk urothelial carcinoma of the upper urinary tract (UUT-UC): Results from a large multicenter collaborative study. *Cancer* **2011**, *117*, 5500–5508. [CrossRef] [PubMed]
7. Browne, B.M.; Stensland, K.D.; Moynihan, M.J.; Canes, D. An Analysis of Staging and Treatment Trends for Upper Tract Urothelial Carcinoma in the National Cancer Database. *Clin. Genitourin. Cancer* **2018**, *16*, e743–e750. [CrossRef] [PubMed]
8. Seisen, T.; Jindal, T.; Karabon, P.; Sood, A.; Bellmunt, J.; Rouprêt, M.; Leow, J.J.; Vetterlein, M.; Sun, M.; Alanee, S.; et al. Efficacy of Systemic Chemotherapy Plus Radical Nephroureterectomy for Metastatic Upper Tract Urothelial Carcinoma. *Eur. Urol.* **2017**, *71*, 714–718. [CrossRef] [PubMed]
9. Moschini, M.; Xylinas, E.; Zamboni, S.; Mattei, A.; Niegisch, G.; Yu, E.Y.; Bamias, A.; Agarwal, N.; Sridhar, S.S.; Sternberg, C.N.; et al. Efficacy of Surgery in the Primary Tumor Site for Metastatic Urothelial Cancer: Analysis of an International, Multicenter, Multidisciplinary Database. *Eur. Urol. Oncol.* **2020**, *3*, 94–101. [CrossRef] [PubMed]

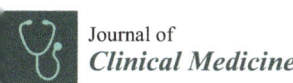

Article

Usefulness of the Urine Methylation Test (Bladder EpiCheck®) in Follow-Up Patients with Non-Muscle Invasive Bladder Cancer and Cytological Diagnosis of Atypical Urothelial Cells—An Institutional Study

Karla B. Peña [1,2,3], Francesc Riu [1,2,3], Anna Hernandez [1,2], Carmen Guilarte [1], Joan Badia [2] and David Parada [1,2,3,*]

1. Molecular Pathology Unit, Department of Pathology, Hospital Universitari de Sant Joan, 43204 Reus, Spain; karlabeatriz.pena@salutsantjoan.cat (K.B.P.); francesc.riu@salutsantjoan.cat (F.R.); anna.hernandez@salutsantjoan.cat (A.H.); carmen.guilarte@salutsantjoan.cat (C.G.)
2. Institut d'Investigació Sanitària Pere Virgili, 43204 Reus, Spain; joan.badia@iispv.cat
3. Facultat de Medicina i Ciències de la Salut, Universitat Rovira i Virgili, 43007 Reus, Spain
* Correspondence: david.parada@urv.cat

Abstract: Urothelial bladder cancer is a heterogeneous disease and one of the most common cancers worldwide. Bladder cancer ranges from low-grade tumors that recur and require long-term invasive surveillance to high-grade tumors with high mortality. After the initial contemporary treatment in non-muscle invasive bladder cancer, recurrence and progression rates remain high. Follow-up of these patients involves the use of cystoscopies, cytology, and imaging of the upper urinary tract in selected patients. However, in this context, both cystoscopy and cytology have limitations. In the follow-up of bladder cancer, the finding of urothelial cells with abnormal cytological characteristics is common. The main objective of our study was to evaluate the usefulness of a urine DNA methylation test in patients with urothelial bladder cancer under follow-up and a cytological finding of urothelial cell atypia. In addition, we analyzed the relationship between the urine DNA methylation test, urine cytology, and subsequent cystoscopy study. It was a prospective and descriptive cohort study conducted on patients presenting with non-muscle invasive urothelial carcinoma between 1 January 2018 and 31 May 2022. A voided urine sample and a DNA methylation test was extracted from each patient. A total of 70 patients, 58 male and 12 female, with a median age of 70.03 years were studied. High-grade urothelial carcinoma was the main histopathological diagnosis. Of the cytologies, 41.46% were cataloged as atypical urothelial cells. The DNA methylation test was positive in 17 urine samples, 51 were negative and 2 were invalid. We demonstrated the usefulness of a DNA methylation test in the follow-up of patients diagnosed with urothelial carcinoma. The methylation test also helps to diagnose urothelial cell atypia.

Keywords: methylation; DNA; urothelial; cancer; bladder; atypia; cytology

Citation: Peña, K.B.; Riu, F.; Hernandez, A.; Guilarte, C.; Badia, J.; Parada, D. Usefulness of the Urine Methylation Test (Bladder EpiCheck®) in Follow-Up Patients with Non-Muscle Invasive Bladder Cancer and Cytological Diagnosis of Atypical Urothelial Cells—An Institutional Study. *J. Clin. Med.* **2022**, *11*, 3855. https://doi.org/10.3390/jcm11133855

Academic Editor: Massimiliano Creta

Received: 21 June 2022
Accepted: 1 July 2022
Published: 3 July 2022

Publisher's Note: MDPI stays neutral with regard to jurisdictional claims in published maps and institutional affiliations.

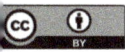

Copyright: © 2022 by the authors. Licensee MDPI, Basel, Switzerland. This article is an open access article distributed under the terms and conditions of the Creative Commons Attribution (CC BY) license (https://creativecommons.org/licenses/by/4.0/).

1. Introduction

Bladder cancer is the tenth most common cancer worldwide, with approximately 573,000 new cases and 213,000 deaths [1,2]. In men, the respective incidence and mortality rates are 9.5 and 3.3 per 100,000 more common than in women [1], and it is the sixth most common cancer and the ninth leading cause of cancer death. In Southern Europe (Greece, Spain and Italy), Western Europe (Belgium and The Netherlands) and North America, the incidence rates are highest for both sexes [1,2].

Bladder cancer is one of the cancers with the longest lifespans and highest costs due to the high rate of recurrence and the need for continuous monitoring [3,4]. Currently, both cystoscopy and urinary cytology are the most common methods of diagnosis in both the detection and the follow-up of malignant urothelial neoplasms [5–8]. However, both methods have advantages and disadvantages. Cystoscopy is an invasive method and causes significant discomfort to patients [5–8], while urinary cytology is non-invasive and effective in diagnosing high-grade (HG) urothelial cancers but has a sensitivity between 11% and 17% to low-grade (LG) urothelial lesions, which are the most common lesions of the bladder [5–8]. Additionally, the consistency and precision of the cytomorphological evaluation may undergo alterations as a consequence of the treatment given for primary or recurrent urothelial neoplasms of the urinary bladder and inflammatory states, which makes a definitive diagnosis difficult [9–12].

Urothelial cells with abnormal cytological characteristics that do not meet the criteria for malignancy are commonly found in the daily practice of urinary cytopathology. In this atypia of urothelial cells, the clinical–cytological correlation is not adequate, and its diagnostic approach remains difficult [13–15]. Various reasons have been given for this: for example, borderline neoplastic urothelial morphological alterations, changes associated with benign processes, such as inflammation, lithiasis, or the effect of local treatment, and even poorly fixed samples [13–18]. Therefore, urinary biomarkers need to be found that can be used in patients with atypical urothelial cells so that they can be studied appropriately. The main objective of our study was to evaluate the usefulness of a urine DNA methylation test in patients with urothelial bladder cancer under follow-up and a cytological finding of urothelial cell atypia. In addition, we analyzed the relationship between the urine DNA methylation test, urine cytology, and subsequent cystoscopy study.

2. Materials and Methods

2.1. Study Design and Patient Cohort

This is a prospective and descriptive cohort study conducted on patients with non-muscle invasive urothelial carcinoma under oncological and urological follow-up at the Urology and Medical Oncology Service of the South Catalonia Oncology Institute (Hospital Universitari de Sant Joan, Reus, Spain), between 1 January 2018 and 31 March 2022. Patients with painless hematuria and Paris system category III, IV, and V, with no histopathological diagnosis were also included (Figure 1). We studied urine samples that 70 patients had submitted to the molecular pathology unit of our pathology department. The patients' clinical data were extracted from medical records and the study was approved by the Institutional Review Board (IISPV). Two urine samples were obtained from each patient simultaneously, one of which was processed for cytological study and the other for DNA methylation study. At the time of evaluating the results of both the cytology study and the methylation test, none of the investigators responsible for the analyses were aware of the results of the tests.

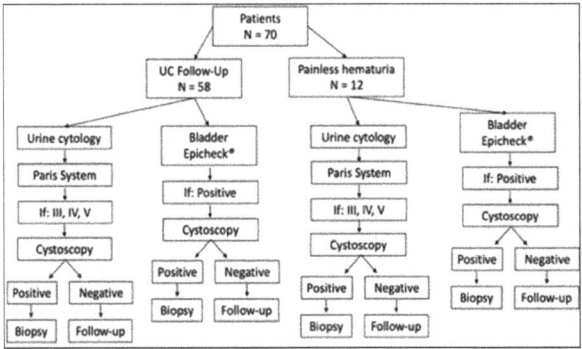

Figure 1. Distribution and workflow for patients included in the present study (N = 70). UC: Urothelial carcinoma.

2.2. Urine Cytology Study

Urine samples were routinely processed with liquid-based cytology using the Thin Prep 5000 TM method (Hologic Co., Marlborough, MA, USA). All the sample material was fixed with the hemolytic and preservative solution Cytolyt™ and spun at 3000 rpm for 5 min. The sediment was then transferred to 20 mL of PreservCyt solution, kept for 15 min at room temperature, and processed with a T5000 automated processor in accordance with the manufacturer's recommendations. One slide was obtained for each sample and fixed in 95% ethanol. The slide was stained with Papanicolaou. All samples were evaluated according to the Paris System to report urine cytology. The diagnostic categories were: category I: insufficient material for diagnosis; category II: negative for high-grade urothelial carcinoma; category III: atypical urothelial cells; category IV: suspicious for high-grade urothelial carcinoma; and category V: high-grade urothelial carcinoma.

2.3. DNA Methylation Study (Bladder EpiCheck® Test)

The Bladder EpiCheck® is an in vitro diagnostic test for the detection of DNA methylation patterns in urine that are associated with bladder cancer. A cell pellet was created from every urine sample for the Bladder EpiCheck® test (Nucleix, Rehovot, Israel). The urine sample was centrifuged twice at $1000 \times g$ for 10 min at room temperature. DNA was extracted from the cell pellet using the Bladder EpiCheck® DNA extraction kit. The extracted DNA was digested using a methylation sensitive restriction enzyme, which cleaves DNA at its recognition sequence if it is unmethylated. The quantitative real-time polymerase chain reaction (qRT-PCR) amplification was performed using Rotor-Gene Q. The samples were prepared for the PCR assay using the Bladder EpiCheck® test kit, and the results were analyzed using the Bladder EpiCheck® software. For samples that pass the internal control validation, the software calculates an EpiScore (between 0 and 100) which represents the overall methylation level of the sample on the panel of biomarkers. The test cut-off is an EpiScore of 60. An EpiScore $\geq$ 60 indicates a high probability of bladder cancer (positive), and a score < 60 indicates a high probability of no bladder cancer or that the cancer is still in remission (negative). An invalid result indicates the test should be repeated.

2.4. Statistical Analysis

Statistical analyses were carried out in "R" (version 4.2.0) using "stats" library (version 4.2.0). Graphs were elaborated in "R" using "ggpubr" and "ggplot2" packages (version 0.4.0 and 3.3.6). Bladder cancer was diagnosed by a pathologist and set as the reference standard against which both urine cytology and bladder epicheck were compared to assess the sensitivity, specificity, positive predictive value and negative predictive. Cytology results were considered negative for categories I and II, atypical for category III and positive for categories IV and V.

3. Results

3.1. Clinical Findings

Our analysis included 58 male and 12 female patients with a median age of 70.02 years (range 49–91 years). In the group under follow-up for urothelial bladder cancer (59 patients), there were 52 males (88.14%) and seven females (11.86%) with a mean age of 71.34 years (range 50–91 years). The previous histopathological diagnosis was carcinoma in situ in six patients (10.17%), high-grade urothelial carcinoma in 37 patients (62.71%), and low-grade urothelial carcinoma in 16 (27.12%) cases. The follow-up time was one year or less in 14 patients (23.73%), between two and five years in 26 patients (44.07%), between six and ten years in 14 patients (23.73%), and more than ten years in five patients (8.47%). Recurrence was observed in 29 patients (49.15%). Thirty-eight (64.40%) patients received intravesical therapy with BCG (see Table 1).

Table 1. Clinical characteristics of patients under investigation for DNA methylation test (N = 70).

Histopathological Diagnosis	LGUC	HGUC	CIS	No Cancer
Patients (N)	16	37	6	11
Age (years) (minimum-maximum)	58–82	50–91	53–65	49–76
Gender				
Male	15	31	6	6
Female	1	6	0	5
Cytological diagnosis (PSC)				
I	5	1	0	0
II	5	11	1	1
III	3	14	4	8
IV	3	10	1	2
V	0	1	0	0
DNA methylation test				
Positive	3	12	2	0
Negative	12	24	4	11
Invalid	1	1	0	0
Primary tumor (Bladder)				
Yes	16	34	6	0
No	0	3	0	11
Cystoscopy				
Positive	3	11	2	0
Negative	11	22	2	5
Unrealized	2	4	2	6
Follow-up time (years)				
<1	1	9	4	10
2–5	10	15	1	1
6–10	4	9	1	0
>10	1	4	0	0
Recurrence				
Yes	11	16	2	11
No	5	21	4	0
Treatment				
BCG	4	28	6	0
Mitomycin	1	0	0	0
Chemotherapy	0	2	0	0
Surgery	1	4	0	0
No	10	3	0	11

PSC: Paris System Category.

3.2. Cytologic Findings

A total of 82 urinary cytologies from 70 patients were analyzed. Of these, six (7.32%) were category I; 25 (30.49%) were category II; 34 (41.46%) were category III; 16 (19.51%) were category IV; and one (1.22%) was category V. The urothelial carcinoma follow-up group contained 71 of these 82 urinary cytologies. In this group, the main diagnostic category was III (21 cytologies), followed by category II (17 cytologies) and category IV (14 cytologies) (Figure 2). In the group with painless hematuria (11), the main diagnostic category was III (8 cytologies), followed by category IV (2 cytologies) and category II (1 cytology) (see Table 1).

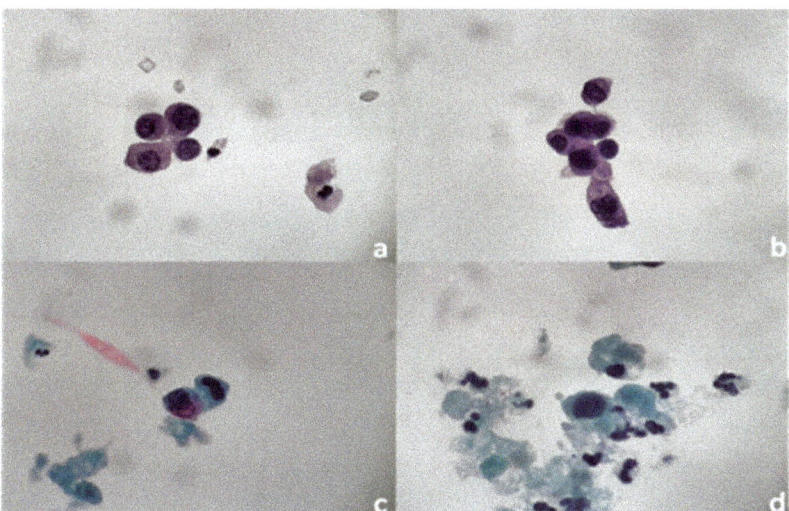

Figure 2. Cytological findings in cases under follow-up for urothelial carcinoma. (**a**) Characteristic finding of atypia urothelial cell. Hyperchromatic nuclei and nuclei/cytoplasm loss. (**b**) Isolated group with evidence of cytologic atypia. Some cytoplasm has a vacuolated aspect with hyperchromatic nuclei. (**c**) Two isolated urothelial cells with marked cytologic atypia suspicious for carcinoma. (**d**) Single urothelial cell with marked loss of nucleus−cytoplasm ratio, nuclear hyperchromatism, and presence of nucleolus. (Papanicolau staining. DA 20× and 40×).

3.3. DNA Methylation Test (Bladder EpiCheck® Test) Findings

In the follow-up urothelial carcinoma group, a total of 71 DNA methylation tests were performed. Two urine tests were invalid for the DNA methylation test. Of the remaining samples, 18 (25.35%) were positive and 51 (71.83%) were negative for the DNA methylation test. In the group with painless hematuria, all samples were negative for the DNA methylation test (see Table 1).

3.4. Relationship between Urinary Cytological Findings and the DNA Methylation Test (Bladder EpiCheck® Test)

For the patients in the urothelial carcinoma group in diagnosis category I (6), the DNA methylation test was negative in five cases and invalid in one. For diagnostic category II (17), the DNA methylation test was negative in 15 cases and positive in two. For diagnostic category III (21), consisting of atypical urothelial cells (AUC), the test was negative in 16 cases and positive in five. In cytological categories IV and V (15), the DNA methylation test was negative in one case, positive in 13 cases and invalid in one. In the painless hematuria group, the DNA methylation test was negative for all the urinary cytologies diagnosed as category II (1), III (8), and IV (2).

The overall sensitivity rates for the DNA methylation test and cytology were 91.67% and 90%, respectively, while the overall specificity rates were 91.89% and 88.89%, respectively. The overall PPV was 81.82% for cytology and 78.57% for the DNA methylation test; the overall NPV was 94.12% for cytology and 97.14% for the DNA methylation test (Table 2, Figure 3).

Table 2. Overall sensitivity, specificity, positive predictive value, and negative predictive value of bladder EpiCheck® and cytology in follow-up non-muscle invasive bladder carcinoma.

	Non-Muscle Invasive Carcinoma	
	Bladder EpiCheck®	Cytology
Sensitivity	91.67%	90%
Specificity	91.89%	88.89%
PPV	78.57%	81.82%
NPV	97.14%	94.12%

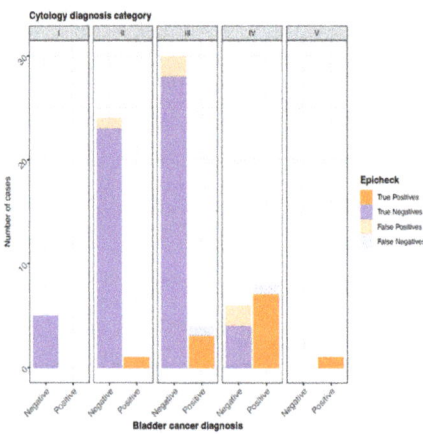

Figure 3. Overall concordance between EpiCheck and bladder diagnosis.

The high-grade urothelial carcinoma sensitivity rates for the DNA methylation test and cytology were 85.71% and 90.91%, respectively, while the specificity rates were 92.31% and 83.33%, respectively. The PPV was 62.50% for the cytology and 70.57% for the DNA methylation test; the NPV was 96.77% for the cytology and 96.77% for the DNA methylation test (Table 3).

Table 3. Sensitivity, specificity, positive predictive value, and negative predictive value of bladder EpiCheck® and cytology in high-grade urothelial carcinoma.

	Non-Muscle Invasive Carcinoma	
	Bladder EpiCheck®	Cytology
Sensitivity	85.71%	90.91%
Specificity	92.31%	83.33%
PPV	70.59%	62.50%
NPV	96.77%	96.77%

4. Discussion

Bladder cancer is mainly diagnosed in the third decade of life [19] and, at the time of diagnosis, patients are in a treatable stage with a long life expectancy but require long periods of surveillance, follow-up, and treatment of recurrences and complications [20,21]. In the urothelial carcinoma group in our study, there was a predominance of males (88.24%), with a mean age of 77.9 years, and more than 80% of the patients had a follow-up time of between one and ten years. [1–4,20,21]. This high recurrence rate of 47.45% evidenced in our study is similar to that described in other publications, in which the recurrence rate can reach 52% at five years, implying a significant prevalence of non-muscle invasive bladder carcinoma (NMIBC). All these data demonstrate a significant burden for the patient and physician, and a high economic impact related to patient care [20,21].

The category of NMIBC includes different types of lesions, such as non-invasive neoplasms, which are those that invade the subepithelial connective tissue and carcinoma in situ. These tumors are frequently treated with different therapeutic options depending on variables such as the histopathological grade and the stage within the clinical context [21]. However, the treatment has the capacity to produce various morphological and cytological alterations that increase the diagnostic difficulty in the follow-up of these patients. For example, it has been described that treatment with immunomodulators such as BCG produces reactive urothelial atypia, in addition to urothelial denudation, granulomatous inflammation, eosinophilic cystitis, and persistence of carcinoma in situ in von Brunn nests [9,10]. In our study, the presence of urothelial atypia was found in 35.59%. In actuality, the rate of notification of urothelial cell atypia ranges between 2 and 31% [22–25]. This greater number of urine cytologies with urothelial atypia in our study could be explained by the changes induced by the treatment administered in our patients.

Currently there are different new urinary biomarkers based on genetic or epigenetic abnormalities that are common in bladder cancer, such as aberrant DNA methylation and non-coding RNA [26–33]. Several of these tests have demonstrated their usefulness in the follow-up of NMIVT patients with very high negative predictive values (NPV) for recurrences of NMIBC (high-grade), which raises the possibility of adapting them to the follow-up of patients [26–31]. In our study, we evaluated the capacity of the DNA methylation test in patients with a cytological diagnosis of urothelial atypia and a cystoscopy study. Thus, the methylation test showed that most of the urothelial atypia cases were negative for the methylation test as well as for the cystoscopy study, which represents a diagnostic aid in this diagnostic category and could be used safely in these patients. In addition, molecular markers can help improve the interpretation capacity of other diagnostic tests, such as urine cytology, through positive feedback. However, additional studies are needed to demonstrate the usefulness of the DNA methylation test in the setting of cytological atypia.

Our analysis of the results of urinary cytology samples and the DNA methylation test showed a reasonable relationship between the negative results of the two methods. In general, the NPV was 96.77% for both the cytology and DNA methylation test in high-grade lesions, but when we analyzed all the lesions, the methylation test showed an value of the NPV, arising to 97.14% and cytology arising to 94.12%. These findings confirm the NPV of the DNA methylation test [34,35]. In addition, molecular markers can help improve the interpretation capacity of other diagnostic tests, such as urine cytology, through positive feedback.

Our study has certain limitations including the small sample size and only six patients having more than one sample evaluated by both cytology and DNA methylation testing; most of our sample had the typical limitation of single visit studies. The inclusion of low-grade urothelial carcinomas can modify the usefulness of the methylation test. However, during the molecular evolution of urothelial carcinoma, 20% of low-grade carcinomas can evolve to high-grade, which is why the test may be useful in monitoring them. Currently, the meaning of the variation in bladder EpiScore values and whether it can provide information on the risk of developing urothelial cancer or response to treatment is unknown.

5. Conclusions

In conclusion, we demonstrate the usefulness of a DNA methylation test in the follow-up of patients diagnosed with urothelial carcinoma and in patients with painless hematuria. The methylation test also helps in the diagnosis of urothelial cell atypia, which involves savings in subsequent clinical studies. New prospective research is needed to define whether the quantitative value of the DNA methylation test can be used as a prognostic factor to predict response to treatment.

Author Contributions: Conceptualization, D.P. and K.B.P.; methodology, D.P., F.R. and A.H.; validation, D.P., J.B. and K.B.P.; formal analysis, D.P. and F.R.; investigation, C.G., A.H. and K.B.P.; resources, D.P., A.H. and F.R.; data curation, D.P. and K.B.P.; writing—original draft preparation, D.P.; writing—review and editing, D.P.; visualization, D.P. and K.B.P.; supervision, D.P. All authors have read and agreed to the published version of the manuscript.

Funding: This research received no external funding.

Institutional Review Board Statement: The study was conducted in accordance with the Declaration of Helsinki and approved by the Institutional Review Board (IISPV) (CEIm: 229/2020).

Informed Consent Statement: Informed consent was obtained from all subjects involved in the study.

Data Availability Statement: All of the data are present in the manuscript.

Acknowledgments: The authors thank John Bates from the linguistic service of the Universitat Rovira I Virgili for his comments and grammar review.

Conflicts of Interest: The authors declare no conflict of interest.

References

1. Sung, H.; Ferlay, J.; Siegel, R.L.; Laversanne, M.; Soerjomataram, I.; Jemal, A.; Bray, F. Global Cancer Statistics 2020: GLOBOCAN Estimates of Incidence and Mortality Worldwide for 36 Cancers in 185 Countries. *CA Cancer J. Clin.* **2021**, *71*, 209–249. [CrossRef] [PubMed]
2. Richters, A.; Aben, K.K.H.; Kiemeney, L.A.L.M. The global burden of urinary bladder cancer: An update. *World J. Urol.* **2020**, *38*, 1895–1904. [CrossRef] [PubMed]
3. Sievert, K.D.; Amend, B.; Nagele, U.; Schilling, D.; Bedke, J.; Horstmann, M.; Hennenlotter, J.; Kruck, S.; Stenzl, A. Economic aspects of bladder cancer: What are the benefits and costs? *World J. Urol.* **2009**, *27*, 295–300. [CrossRef] [PubMed]
4. Sloan, F.A.; Yashkin, A.P.; Akushevich, I.; Inman, B.A. The Cost to Medicare of Bladder Cancer Care. *Eur. Urol. Oncol.* **2020**, *3*, 515–522. [CrossRef] [PubMed]
5. Wiener, H.G.; Mian, C.; Haitel, A.; Pycha, A.; Schatzl, G.; Marberger, M. Can urine bound diagnostic tests replace cystoscopy in the management of bladder cancer? *J. Urol.* **1998**, *159*, 1876–1880. [CrossRef]
6. Leyh, H.; Marberger, M.; Conort, P.; Sternberg, C.; Pansadoro, V.; Pagano, F.; Bassi, P.; Boccon-Gibod, L.; Ravery, V.; Treiber, U.; et al. Comparison of the BTA stat test with voided urine cytology and bladder wash cytology in the diagnosis and monitoring of bladder cancer. *Eur. Urol.* **1999**, *35*, 52–56. [CrossRef] [PubMed]
7. Van Rhijn, B.W.; van der Poel, H.G.; van der Kwast, T.H. Urine markers for bladder cancer surveillance: A systematic review. *Eur. Urol.* **2005**, *47*, 736–748. [CrossRef]
8. Hentschel, A.E.; van der Toom, E.E.; Vis, A.N.; Ket, J.C.F.; Bosschieter, J.; Heymans, M.W.; van Moorselaar, R.J.A.; Steenbergen, R.D.M.; Nieuwenhuijzen, J.A. A systematic review on mutation markers for bladder cancer diagnosis in urine. *BJU Int.* **2021**, *127*, 12–27. [CrossRef]
9. Lopez-Beltran, A.; Paner, G.P.; Montironi, R.; Raspollini, M.R.; Cheng, L. Iatrogenic changes in the urinary tract. *Histopathology* **2017**, *70*, 10–25. [CrossRef]
10. Lopez-Beltran, A.; Montironi, R.; Raspollini, M.R.; Cheng, L.; Netto, G.J. Iatrogenic pathology of the urinary bladder. *Semin. Diagn. Pathol.* **2018**, *35*, 218–227. [CrossRef]
11. Cakir, E.; Kucuk, U.; Pala, E.E.; Sezer, O.; Ekin, R.G.; Cakmak, O. Cytopathologic differential diagnosis of low-grade urothelial carcinoma and reactive urothelial proliferation in bladder washings: A logistic regression analysis. *APMIS* **2017**, *125*, 431–436. [CrossRef] [PubMed]
12. Sanfrancesco, J.; Jones, J.S.; Hansel, D.E. Diagnostically challenging cases: What are atypia and dysplasia? *Urol. Clin. N. Am.* **2013**, *40*, 281–293. [CrossRef] [PubMed]
13. Brimo, F.; Vollmer, R.T.; Case, B.; Aprikian, A.; Kassouf, W.; Auger, M. Accuracy of urine cytology and the significance of an atypical category. *Am. J. Clin. Pathol.* **2009**, *132*, 785–793. [CrossRef] [PubMed]
14. Bostwick, D.G.; Hossain, D. Does subdivision of the "atypical" urine cytology increase predictive accuracy for urothelial carcinoma? *Diagn. Cytopathol.* **2014**, *42*, 1034–1044. [CrossRef] [PubMed]
15. Chau, K.; Rosen, L.; Coutsouvelis, C.; Fenelus, M.; Brenkert, R.; Klein, M.; Stone, G.; Raab, S.; Aziz, M.; Cocker, R. Accuracy and risk of malignancy for diagnostic categories in urine cytology at a large tertiary institution. *Cancer Cytopathol.* **2015**, *123*, 10–18. [CrossRef]
16. Raab, S.S.; Lenel, J.C.; Cohen, M.B. Low grade transitional cell carcinoma of the bladder. Cytologic diagnosis by key features as identified by logistic regression analysis. *Cancer* **1994**, *74*, 1621–1626. [CrossRef]
17. Bhatia, A.; Dey, P.; Kakkar, N.; Srinivasan, R.; Nijhawan, R. Malignant atypical cell in urine cytology: A diagnostic dilemma. *Cytojournal* **2006**, *3*, 28. [CrossRef]

18. Mokhtar, G.A.; Al-Dousari, M.; Al-Ghamedi, D. Diagnostic significance of atypical category in the voided urine samples: A retrospective study in a tertiary care center. *Urol. Ann.* **2010**, *2*, 100–106. [CrossRef]
19. Madeb, R.; Messing, E.M. Gender, racial and age differences in bladder cancer incidence and mortality. *Urol. Oncol.* **2004**, *22*, 86–92. [CrossRef]
20. Sloan, F.A.; Yashkin, A.P.; Akushevich, I.; Inman, B.A. Longitudinal patterns of cost and utilization of medicare beneficiaries with bladder cancer. *Urol. Oncol.* **2020**, *38*, e11–e39. [CrossRef]
21. Witjes, J.A. Follow-up in non-muscle invasive bladder cancer: Facts and future. *World J. Urol.* **2021**, *39*, 4047–4053. [CrossRef] [PubMed]
22. Layfield, L.J.; Elsheikh, T.M.; Fili, A.; Nayar, R.; Shidham, V.; Papanicolaou Society of Cytopathology. Review of the state of the art and recommendations of the Papanicolaou Society of Cytopathology for urinary cytology procedures and reporting: The Papanicolaou Society of Cytopathology Practice Guidelines Task Force. *Diagn. Cytopathol.* **2004**, *30*, 24–30. [CrossRef] [PubMed]
23. Mikou, P.; Lenos, M.; Papaioannou, D.; Vrettou, K.; Trigka, E.A.; Sousouris, S.; Constantinides, C. Evaluation of the Paris System in atypical urinary cytology. *Cytopathology* **2018**, *29*, 545–549. [CrossRef]
24. Barkan, G.; Elsheikh, T.; Kurtycz, D.; Minamiguchi, S.; Ohtani, H.; Piaton, E.; Savic, S.; Tabatabai, Z.; VandenBussche, C. Atypical Urothelial Cells (AUC). In *The Paris System for Reporting Urinary Cytology*, 1st ed.; Dorothy, L., Rosenthal, A., Eva, M., Wojcik, B., Daniel, F.I., Kurtycz, C., Eds.; Springer: New York, NY, USA, 2016; pp. 39–48.
25. Granados, R.; Duarte, J.A.; Corrales, T.; Camarmo, E.; Bajo, P. Applying the Paris System for Reporting Urine Cytology Increases the Rate of Atypical Urothelial Cells in Benign Cases: A Need for Patient Management Recommendations. *Acta Cytol.* **2017**, *61*, 71–76. [CrossRef] [PubMed]
26. Santoni, G.; Morelli, M.B.; Amantini, C.; Battelli, N. Urinary Markers in Bladder Cancer: An Update. *Front. Oncol.* **2018**, *8*, 362. [CrossRef] [PubMed]
27. Maas, M.; Walz, S.; Stühler, V.; Aufderklamm, S.; Rausch, S.; Bedke, J.; Stenzl, A.; Todenhöfer, T. Molecular markers in disease detection and follow-up of patients with non-muscle invasive bladder cancer. *Expert Rev. Mol. Diagn.* **2018**, *18*, 443–455. [CrossRef] [PubMed]
28. Porten, S.P. Epigenetic Alterations in Bladder Cancer. *Curr. Urol. Rep.* **2018**, *19*, 102. [CrossRef]
29. Li, H.T.; Duymich, C.E.; Weisenberger, D.J.; Liang, G. Genetic and Epigenetic Alterations in Bladder Cancer. *Int. Neurourol. J.* **2016**, *20* (Suppl. S2), S84–S94. [CrossRef]
30. D'Andrea, D.; Soria, F.; Zehetmayer, S.; Gust, K.M.; Korn, S.; Witjes, J.A.; Shariat, S.F. Diagnostic accuracy, clinical utility and influence on decision-making of a methylation urine biomarker test in the surveillance of non-muscle-invasive bladder cancer. *BJU Int.* **2019**, *123*, 959–967. [CrossRef]
31. Trenti, E.; D'Elia, C.; Mian, C.; Schwienbacher, C.; Hanspeter, E.; Pycha, A.; Kafka, M.; Degener, S.; Danuser, H.; Roth, S.; et al. Diagnostic predictive value of the Bladder EpiCheck test in the follow-up of patients with non-muscle-invasive bladder cancer. *Cancer Cytopathol.* **2019**, *127*, 465–469. [CrossRef]
32. Huang, H.M.; Li, H.X. Tumor heterogeneity and the potential role of liquid biopsy in bladder cancer. *Cancer Commun.* **2021**, *41*, 91–108. [CrossRef] [PubMed]
33. Crocetto, F.; Barone, B.; Ferro, M.; Busetto, G.M.; La Civita, E.; Buonerba, C.; Di Lorenzo, G.; Terracciano, D.; Schalken, J.A. Liquid biopsy in bladder cancer: State of the art and future perspectives. *Crit. Rev. Oncol. Hematol.* **2022**, *170*, 103577. [CrossRef] [PubMed]
34. Pierconti, F.; Martini, M.; Fiorentino, V.; Cenci, T.; Capodimonti, S.; Straccia, P.; Sacco, E.; Pugliese, D.; Cindolo, L.; Larocca, L.M.; et al. The combination cytology/epichek test in non muscle invasive bladder carcinoma follow-up: Effective tool or useless expence? *Urol. Oncol.* **2021**, *39*, e17–e131. [CrossRef] [PubMed]
35. Cochetti, G.; Rossi de Vermandois, J.A.; Maulà, V.; Cari, L.; Cagnani, R.; Suvieri, C.; Balducci, P.M.; Paladini, A.; Del Zingaro, M.; Nocentini, G.; et al. Diagnostic performance of the Bladder EpiCheck methylation test and photodynamic diagnosis-guided cystoscopy in the surveil-lance of high-risk non-muscle invasive bladder cancer: A single centre, prospective, blinded clinical trial. *Urol. Oncol.* **2022**, *40*, 105.e11–105.e18. [CrossRef]

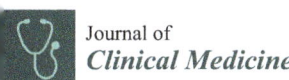 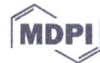

Review

A Systematic Review on the Role of Repeat Transurethral Resection after Initial en Bloc Resection for Non-Muscle Invasive Bladder Cancer

Henglong Hu [1], Mengqi Zhou [1,2], Binrui Yang [1,2], Shiwei Zhou [1,2], Zheng Liu [1] and Jiaqiao Zhang [1,*]

[1] Department of Urology, Institute of Urology, Tongji Hospital, Tongji Medical College, Huazhong University of Science and Technology, No. 1095 Jiefang Avenue, Wuhan 430030, China
[2] College of Life Science and Technology, Huazhong University of Science and Technology, 1037 Luoyu Road, Wuhan 430074, China
* Correspondence: medzjq@hust.edu.cn; Tel.: +86-027-8366-5307

Abstract: International guidelines recommend repeat transurethral resection of bladder tumors (reTURB) for selected patients with high-risk non-muscle invasive bladder cancer to remove possible residual tumors, restage tumors and improve the therapeutic outcome. However, most evidence supporting the benefits of reTURB is from conventional TURB. The role of reTURB in patients receiving initial En bloc resection of bladder tumor (ERBT) is still unknown. PubMed, Embase, Web of Science, The Cochrane Library, and China National Knowledge Infrastructure (CNKI) were systematically searched. Finally, this systematic review and meta-analysis included twelve articles, including 539 patients. The rates of residual tumor and tumor upstaging detected by reTURB after ERBT were 5.9% (95%CI, 2.0–11.1%) and 0.0% (95%CI, 0.0–0.5%), respectively. Recurrence-free survival, tumor recurrence and progression were comparable between patients with and without reTURB after initial ERBT. The pooled hazard ratios of 1-year, 2-year, 3-year and 5-year recurrence-free survival were 0.74 (95%CI, 0.36–1.51; $p = 0.40$), 0.76 (95%CI, 0.45–1.26; $p = 0.28$), 0.83 (95%CI, 0.53–1.32; $p = 0.43$) and 0.83 (95%CI, 0.56–1.23; $p = 0.36$), respectively. The pooled relative risks of recurrence and progression were 0.87 (95%CI, 0.64–1.20; $p = 0.40$) and 1.11 (95%CI, 0.54–2.32; $p = 0.77$), respectively. Current evidence demonstrates that reTURB after ERBT for bladder cancer can detect relatively low rates of residual tumor and tumor upstaging and appears not to improve either recurrence or progression.

Keywords: bladder cancer; repeat transurethral resection; re-resection; restage; en bloc resection; systematic review

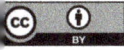

1. Introduction

Bladder cancer is among the world's top ten most common cancer types, with approximately 550,000 new cases annually [1,2]. Non-muscle-invasive bladder cancer (NMIBC), which includes Ta, T1, and carcinoma in situ, represents approximately 75% of all bladder cancers at initial diagnosis [3]. Transurethral resection of the bladder (TURB) is the standard procedure for bladder cancer diagnosis and represents, at the same time, the most important therapeutic moment for patients with NMIBC [3]. Although conventional TURB (cTURB) is widely used and has piled tremendous expertise over decades, multiple drawbacks are still associated with it. Such issues are, for example, tumor cell scattering through fragmentation, the risk of tumor cell seeding and reimplantation, a rather high rate of missing detrusor muscle (DM) and downstaging, thermal damage of sensitive areas within the specimens, and incomplete resections [4].

To overcome these drawbacks of cTURB, En bloc resection of bladder tumor (ERBT) and second or repeat TURB (reTURB) have been introduced to clinical practice [4]. ERBT applies a novel technique to cTURB, resecting the entire tumor, the surrounding mucosa, the underlying stroma, and superficial muscularis propria in a single specimen [5]. Recently, there has been increasing evidence to support the clinical benefit of ERBT. Compared to cTURB, ERBT has a higher DM presence rate, seems safer, and yields superior histopathologic information and performance [6,7]. ERBT is most feasible for patients with bladder tumor size of ≤3 cm. For bladder tumor size of >3 cm, the specimen may not be retrieved in one piece. However, the resection procedure itself is still technically possible, and the potential benefits can still be preserved [8].

An early reTURB is recommended to be performed for selected patients by all the most followed international guidelines in the urological community (Table 1) [3,9–15]. Compared with initial TURB, reTURB can remove the residual tumors, detect understaging BC, improve the responsive rate of intravesical Bacillus Calmette-Guerin (BCG) instillation, and instruct further treatments [16–19]. A recent study corroborated the important role of routine reTURB, followed by an adequate maintenance course of BCG in organ-sparing NMIBC patients [20]. Interestingly, reTURB was found to be associated with longer recurrence-free survival (RFS) in patients receiving TICE strain maintenance therapy than those using Connaught and RIVM [20,21]. However, it should be underlined that reTURB, which must be done on a patient who may still be suffering from the consequences of the last surgery, is an invasive and morbid technique that significantly lowers the patient quality of life. In addition, it increases the economic burden of bladder cancer care [22]. Moreover, there is no complete agreement in international guidelines as to which patients should be recommended for reTURB surgery, and these recommendations do not consider the impact of the surgical approach (Table 1) [3,9–14]. That is why we must further clarify which patients benefit most from reTURB. Currently, most evidence supporting the benefits of reTURB is based on patients receiving previous cTURB [17]. Whether reTURB can improve the outcomes of patients receiving initial ERBT and whether reTURB can be safely avoided by ERBT patients is still unclear. Therefore, we set out to perform this systematic review and meta-analysis.

Table 1. ReTURB recommendations across international guideline panels.

Guidelines Body	Version	Recommendation on Suitable reTURB Candidates	Recommendation Strength	ReTURB Period after the Initial Resection
European Association of Urology	2022	1. Incomplete initial TURB, or in case of doubt about the completeness of a TURB; 2. If there is no detrusor muscle in the specimen after initial resection, except for Ta LG/G1 tumors and primary CIS; 3. T1 tumors.	Strong	2–6 weeks
National Comprehensive Cancer Network (NCCN)	Version 2.2022	1. Visually incomplete resection or **high-volume tumor** 2. **TaHG, particularly if large**, and/or no muscle in the specimen 3. T1 tumors	2A *	2–6 weeks
European Society for Medical Oncology (ESMO)	2021	1. The initial TURB was incomplete. 2. If no detrusor muscle exists in the specimen on the initial resection, except for Ta LG and CIS. 3. In all pT1 tumors and **all HG tumors, except for patients with primary CIS**	Strong	4–6 weeks
Canadian Urological Association	2021	1. Incomplete initial TURB 2. **TaHG tumors (e.g., large and/or multiple tumors)** 3. T1 tumors	1. Strong 2. Weak 3. Strong	within 6 weeks
American Urological Association & Society of Urological Oncology	2020	1. Incomplete initial TURB 2. **TaHG tumors** 3. T1 tumors	1. Strong 2. Moderate 3. Strong	within 6 weeks
Chinese Urological Association	2019	1. Incomplete initial TURB 2. No muscle in specimen except for Ta LG/Gl and primary CIS 3. T1 tumors.	Moderate	2–6 weeks

Table 1. *Cont.*

Guidelines Body	Version	Recommendation on Suitable reTURB Candidates	Recommendation Strength	ReTURB Period after the Initial Resection
SIU & International Consultation on Bladder Cancer (ICUD) 2017	2017	1. Incomplete initial resection 2. **TaHG tumors, particularly for patients with large or multifocal tumors** 3. T1 disease	1. B ** 2. C ** 3. B **	within 6 weeks
National Institute for Clinical Excellence (NICE)	2015	1. **All high-risk non-muscle invasive bladder cancer**	1. Low	within 6 weeks

The bold text represents the differences from EAU guidelines. TURB: transurethral resection of bladder tumor; CIS carcinoma in situ; LG: low grade; HG: high grade; * NCCN Categories of Evidence and Consensus; ** recommendation grades of Oxford Centre for Evidence-based Medicine.

2. Materials and Methods

2.1. Literature Search and Study Selection

The Preferred Reporting Items for Systematic Reviews and Meta-Analyses (PRISMA) statement was followed by our study [23]. The protocol of this study has been registered in Open Science Framework Registry (Registration DOI:10.17605/OSF.IO/9FWVM). PubMed, Embase, Web of Science, The Cochrane Library, and China National Knowledge Infrastructure (CNKI) were systematically searched to identify relevant studies. The search was first performed on 30 April 2022 and updated on 12 July 2022. The initial search process was designed to find all relevant published original articles without limitation by year or language. Detailed search terms were: (repeat* [Title/Abstract] OR second [Title/Abstract] OR re-resect* [Title/Abstract] OR re-transurethral [Title/Abstract] OR restag* [Title/Abstract] OR reTUR* [Title/Abstract] OR re-look [Title/Abstract]) AND ("en bloc" [Title/Abstract] OR "en-bloc" [Title/Abstract] OR "enbloc" [Title/Abstract] OR "ERBT" [Title/Abstract] OR enucleate* [Title/Abstract] OR "one piece" [Title/Abstract]) AND ("bladder cancer" [Title/Abstract] OR "bladder tumor" [Title/Abstract] OR "bladder carcinoma" [Title/Abstract] OR "Urothelial carcinoma" [Title/Abstract]). Initial screening was performed independently by two investigators (Dr. Henglong Hu and Dr. Jiaqiao Zhang) based on the titles and abstracts to identify eligible reports. Potentially relevant reports were subjected to a full-text review. Disagreements were resolved by consensus with the co-investigators.

2.2. Inclusion and Exclusion Criteria

We focused on the reTURB outcomes after ERBT, such as residual tumors, upstage, short-term or long-term recurrence and progression. All kinds of study designs, such as randomized control trials (RCTs), cohort studies and single-arm studies, would be included as long as they reported at least one of the interesting outcomes. However, studies lacking original or necessary data, reviews, letters, conference abstracts, editorial materials, replies from authors, case reports, and patent records were excluded. Studies were excluded if the number of participants was less than five, as they were deemed methodologically inappropriate. In cases of duplicate publications or duplicate data, the study of higher quality or the most recent publication was selected. Disagreements were resolved through discussions.

2.3. Data Extraction and Study Quality Assessment

Two investigators extracted the following data from each eligible study independently: first author's name, publication journal and year, countries, study design, study period, sample size, participants' characteristics (age, gender), tumor characteristics, en bloc method, reTURB criteria, intravesical therapy, perioperative complications, recurrence and progression status, recurrence-free survival (RFS), progression-free survival (PFS), overall survival (OS) and cancer-specific survival (CSS). Disagreements between the two authors will be resolved by rechecking the articles and discussion. The methodological quality of cohort studies was evaluated using the Newcastle-Ottawa Scale (NOS) for non-randomized controlled trials [24]. The NOS comprises three domains, including participant selection (points range: 0–4), comparability between groups (points range: 0–2), and clinical outcomes (points range: 0–3). NOS scores ≥ 6 indicate high methodological quality. For single-arm studies and studies in which we only retrieved one arm data, a five-criterion quality appraisal checklist proposed by the European Association of Urology Guidelines Office was used [25]. The five aspects included: 1. Was there an a priori protocol? 2. Was the total population included or were study participants selected consecutively? 3. Was outcome data complete for all participants, and was any missing data adequately explained/unlikely to be related to the outcome? 4. Were all prespecified outcomes of interest and expected outcomes reported? 5. Were primary benefit and harm outcomes appropriately measured? If the answer to all five questions is "yes," the study is at a "low" risk of bias. If the answer to any question is "no", the study is at a "high" risk of bias [25]. Possible publication bias was assessed using funnel plots, Egger test, and Begg's test.

2.4. Data Processing and Statistical Analysis

Dichotomous variables were reported by counts and percentages, while continuous variables were reported as mean± standard difference or median ± interquartile range (IQR: 25th and 75th) or range. The impact of reTURB on survival and disease control was measured by the effect size of the hazard ratio (HR), RFS, PFS, OS, and CSS. They were extracted directly from each study if reported by the authors. Otherwise, these data were estimated indirectly using the method described by Tierney et al. [26]. Each study's Kaplan–Meier plots were downloaded and digitized using the GetData Graph Digitizer (version 2.26; http://getdata-graph-digitizer.com/index.php; accessed on 1 July 2022), and survival probabilities at different follow-up times were extracted. Then, the number of subjects at risk, adjusted for censoring at different follow-up times, was calculated to reconstruct the HR estimate.

The statistical analysis and meta-analysis were performed using STATA version 17.0 software (StataCorp, College Station, TX, USA). A p-value less than 0.05 was considered statistically significant. Heterogeneity among studies was evaluated by the chi-square test, I^2 statistics, and Galbraith plots. Moreover, the pooled estimates were calculated with the fixed-effect model if no significant heterogeneity was detected; otherwise, the random-effect model was used. The z-test determined the pooled effects. As mentioned above, funnel plots were generated to assess any bias, and both the Egger and Begg's tests were done to examine any statistical significance of publication bias. If there is a significant publication bias or pooled studies of less than five, a sensitivity analysis was performed using the trim and fill method to test the robustness of the results.

3. Results
3.1. Literature Search and Study Selection

Figure 1 shows the process of literature search and study selection. Electronic searches of five databases revealed 214 records. After screening titles and abstracts, we found 25 articles relevant to the study aim, and therefore we retrieved the full-text articles. After full-text analysis, another 13 studies were excluded for the following reasons: nine lacked necessary data, two reported duplicated data, and only two studies only reported one patient. Finally, 12 studies fulfilled our eligibility criteria and were enrolled in this review [27–38].

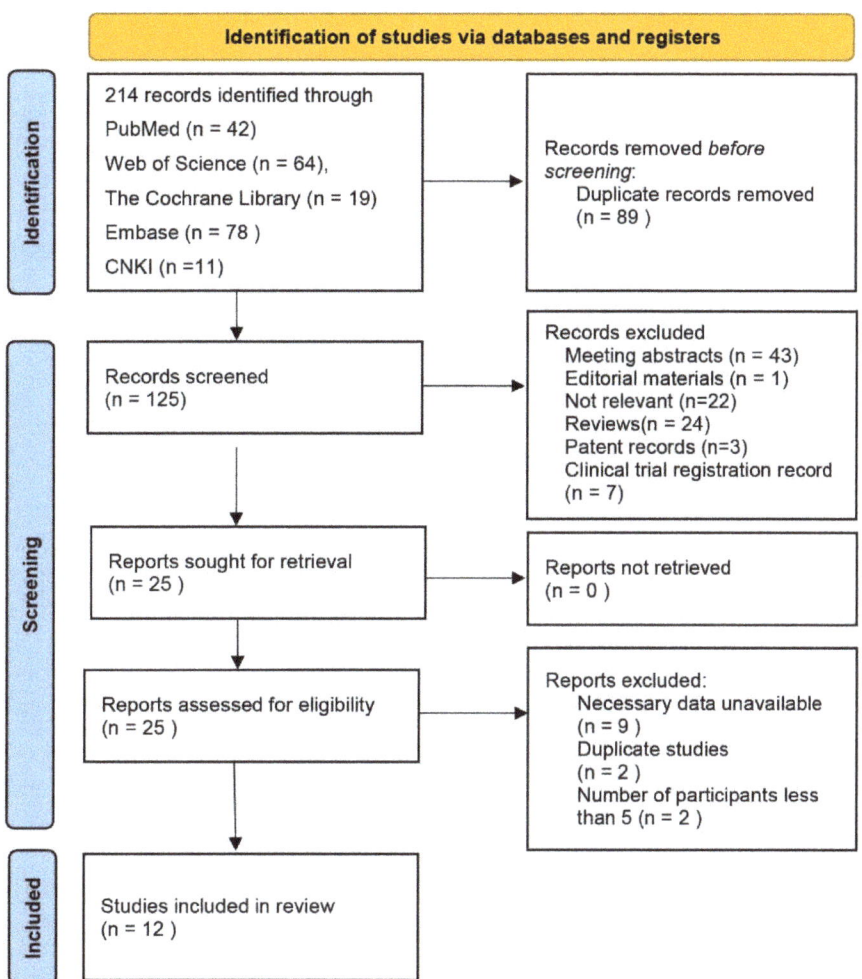

Figure 1. Flowchart of the studies selection process. CNKI: China national knowledge infrastructure.

3.2. Systematic Reviews of Included Studies

Table 2 summarizes the characteristics of the 12 eligible studies published from 2011 to 2022. Five of the studies were conducted in China [31,32,34,36,37], three in Italy [28–30] and one each in Egypt [33], Germany [27], Japan [38], and Poland [35]. All these studies were conducted in the last 12 years. Most patients included were high-risk patients with high-grade and/or tumors. Some studies had limited the tumor size to less than 3 cm or 4 cm. Some early studies only included single tumor patients to facilitate the en bloc resection, and recent studies had no limits or limited the neoplasm number to no more than 3 or 4. The re-resection time was relatively consistent, most of them were performed within 6 weeks after the initial resection. There are three cohort studies that directly compared patients who received reTURB after ERBT with those who only underwent ERBT [32,36,38]. All these studies were published in the last two years which indicates that this topic has recently gained the attention of researchers and is gradually becoming popular. There are six single arm studies that reported the outcome of reTURB after ERBT. Although the objectives of two cohort studies and one RCT were to compare ERBT with cTURB, the data of the ERBT arm of the three studies were also retrieved and analyzed.

Table 2. Characteristics and outcomes of included studies.

First Author & Year	Country	Study Type	Study Period	ReTURB Time	Participants	Groups	Patient Number	Male/Female	Age Mean ± SD (Range) /Median (IQR)	Stage Ta/T1/Tis	Grade LG/HG	Residual Tumor (%)	Up Stage (%)	Recurrence (%)	RFS	Progression	PFS
Zhou 2020 [5]	China	RC	June 2012–June 2018	Within 2–6 weeks	Primary T1 and HG/G3 tumors, excluding primary CIS	ReTURB	108	86/22	66.12 ± 1.52	60/48/0	25/83	6 (5.6)	2 (1.85)	23 (21.3)	1 year: 92.6 2 year: 88.4 * 3 year: 84.3 5 year: 68.0 *	4 (3.7)	1 year: 98.1 3 year: 96.3
						Control	143	111/32	68.59 ± 1.36	87/56/0	49/94	11 (7.69)	2 (1.40)	39 (27.2)	1 year: 90.2 2 year: 84.2 * 3 year: 80.4 5 year: 54.1 *	7 (4.9)	1 year: 97.9 3 year: 95.1
Xu 2021 [26]	China	RC	June 2015–June 2019	Within 6 weeks	Primary T1/TaHG tumors, Tumor number ≤ 4 Diameter ≤ 4 cm	ReTURB	51	41/10	67.4 ± 9.5	16/35/0	13/38	3 (5.88)	0 (0)	10 (19.6)	1 year: 92.2 2 year: 87.6 * 3 year: 81.1 * 5 year: 71.5 *	2 (3.9)	NA
						Control	64	53/11	66.8 ± 9.0	15/49/0	10/54	2 (3.13)	0 (0)	18 (28.1)	1 year: 90.6 2 year: 81.1 * 3 year: 66.4 * 5 year: 63.1 *	1 (1.5)	NA
Yanagisawa 2022 [8]	Japan	RC	April 2013–February 2021	Within 2–6 weeks	T1 Tumors	ReTURB	50	33/17	74 (70,25–78)	0/50/0	0/50	9 (18.0)	0 (0)	18 (36.0)	1 year: 66.5 * 2 year: 55.1 3 year: 54.9 * 5 year: 54.9 *	7 (14.0)	1 year: 95.7 3 year: 80.6 5 year: 64.5 *
						Control	56	43/13	76 (69–82,25)	0/56/0	0/56	NA	NA	18 (32.1)	1 year: 71.3 * 2 year: 59.9 3 year: 59.9 * 5 year: 54.0 *	6 (10.7)	1 year: 95.7 3 year: 82.6 5 year: 82.6 *
Wolters 2011 [27]	Germany	CS	June 2010–October 2010	Within 6 weeks	Solitary papillary lesions, treatment-naive, on the lower bladder wall and trigonum	ReTURB	5	4/1	57 (57–80)	2/3/0	G1 1 G2 1 G3 3	NA	NA	NA	NA	NA	NA
Muto 2014 [28]	Italy	PCS	April 2011–September 2012	Within 30–90 days	Naïve NMIBC	ReTURB	48	NA	NA	31/17/0	31/17/0	0 (0)	0 (0)	7 (14.6)	1.5 year: 85.4	0 (0)	NA

Table 2. *Cont.*

First Author & Year	Country	Study Type	Study Period	ReTURB Time	Participants	Groups	Patient Number	Male/Female	Age Mean ± SD (Range)/Median (IQR)	Stage Ta/T1/Tis	Grade LG/HG	Residual Tumor (%)	Up Stage (%)	Recurrence (%)	RFS	Progression	PFS
Migliari 2015 [26]	Italy	PC	February 2012–September 2013	Within 90 days	Single papillary bladder tumor, diameter ≥ 1 cm	ReTURB	53	NA	NA	30/23/0	30/23	0 (0)	0 (0)	12 (22.6)	1.5 year: Ta 90.0 T1 76.0	0 (0)	NA
Hurle 2020 [30]	Italy	RCS	September 2011–April 2017	Within 40 days	First diagnosis or a primary recurrence of High-risk NMIBC, a single tumor of ≤3 cm and ≤4 lesions	ReTURB	78	51/27	68 ± 9	17/57/4	G3-72	5 (6.41)	0 (0)	11 (14.1)	1 year: 93.4 * 2 year: 92.0 * 3 year: 85.0 * 5 year: 85.0 *	1 (1.3)	NA
Yang 2020 [31]	China	PC	October 2015–June 2017	Within 2–6 weeks	Primary, HG and/or T1 tumor, diameter between 1.0 to 3.0 cm	ReTURB	28	NA	NA	NA	NA	2 (7.14)	1 (3.57)	NA	NA	NA	NA
Hashem 2021 [32]	Egypt	RCT	September 2015–September 2018	4 weeks after the primary resection	NMIBC	ReTURB	44	NA	NA	2/42	28/16	3 (6.82)	0 (0)	7 (15.9)	1 year: 92.6 * 2 year: 80.0 * 3 year: 80.0 *	NA	NA
Hu 2021 [34]	China	RCS	January 2019–October 2019	4–6 weeks	Primary T1 or TaHG	ReTURB	10	NA	NA	NA	NA	0 (0)	0 (0)	NA	NA	NA	NA
Poletajew 2021 [35]	Poland	PC	NA	Within 2–6 weeks	1–4 cm in diameter	ReTURB	37	NA	NA	NA	NA	11 (29.73)	NA	NA	NA	NA	NA
Fan 2022 [37]	China	RCS	2013–2019	Within 6 weeks	NA	ReTURB	27	NA	NA	NA	NA	4 (14.81)	NA	NA	NA	NA	NA

CS: case series; HG: high grade; IQR: interquartile range; LG: low grade; NA: not available; NMIBC: non-muscle invasive bladder cancer; PC: prospective cohort; PCS: prospective case series; RC: retrospective cohort; RCS: retrospective case series; reTURB: repeat transurethral resection of bladder tumor; RFS: recurrence-free survival; PFS: progression-free survival; SD: standard deviation; * Digitized from the Kaplan–Meier plots.

3.3. Residual Tumors and Upstage at reTURB after ERBT

All 12 studies reported the status of residual tumor after ERBT. The residual tumor rate varied from 0% to 29.3%. As shown in Figure 2A, pooling the data from 539 patients demonstrated that the residual tumor rate detected by reTURB after ERBT was 5.9% (95%CI, 2.0–11.1%). Only one study reported the residual tumor location [38]. Among 50 patients, six had residual tumors at the original site, while two were at the non-original site. Ten studies revealed the upstaging rate at reTURB after ERBT ranged from 0% to 3.57%. Surprisingly, as shown in Figure 2B, the meta-analysis demonstrated that the upstaging rate at reTURB is 0.0% (95%CI, 0.0–0.5%).

3.4. Recurrence and Progression

Table 2 provides the recurrence, progression, RFS, and PFS data. The recurrence rate ranges from 14.1% to 36.0% in the reTURB group and 27.2% to 32.1% in the patients who did not receive reTURB. RFS was comparable between patients with and without reTURB after initial ERBT. The pooled HRs of 1-year, 2-year, 3-year and 5-year RFS were 0.74 (95%CI, 0.36–1.51; $p = 0.40$), 0.76 (95%CI, 0.45–1.26; $p = 0.28$), 0.83 (95%CI, 0.53–1.32; $p = 0.43$) and 0.83 (95%CI, 0.56–1.23; $p = 0.36$), respectively (Figure 3). The pooled relative risk (RR) of recurrence was 0.87 (95%CI, 0.64–1.20; $p = 0.40$) (Figure 4A). The progression rate ranged from 0.0% to 14.0% in the reTURB group and 1.5% to 10.7% in the control group. Meta-analysis reveals that RR of progression was 1.11 (95%CI, 0.54–2.32; $p = 0.77$) (Figure 4B). No study reported the outcomes of OS and CSS.

3.5. Risk of Bias Assessment, Heterogeneity, and Sensitivity Analysis

The NOS scores of three cohort studies have been shown in Table S1, and the quality of these three studies was considered high. All the other studies except for the RCT article have been assessed by the five-criterion quality appraisal checklist and consider to be at high risk of bias (Table S2). Heterogeneity among comparative studies was evaluated by the chi-square test, I^2 statistics, and Galbraith plots (Figure 5). No significant heterogeneity was detected. Although no significant publication bias was found in the funnel plot (Figure 6), Egger test, and Begg's test (Table S3). We also performed a sensitivity analysis. The sensitivity analysis using the trim and fill method generated similar results, which indicated these pooling results were stable and reliable (Table S3). Figure S1 shows the funnel plots of sensitivity analysis.

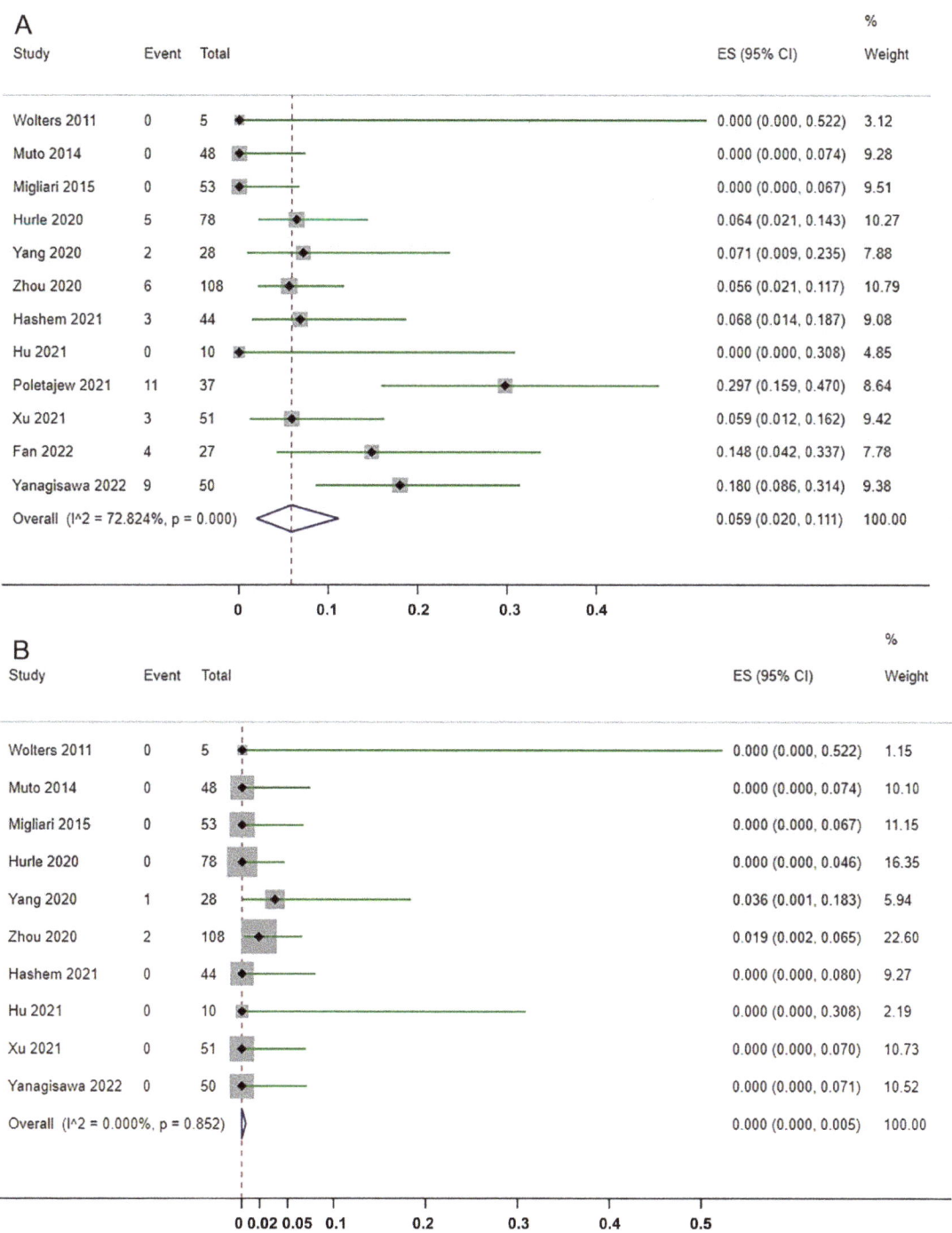

Figure 2. Forest plots of the rates of residual tumor (**A**) and tumor upstaging (**B**) detected by reTURB after initial ERBT [27–38]. ES: effect size. The dash lines represent the pooled effect size.

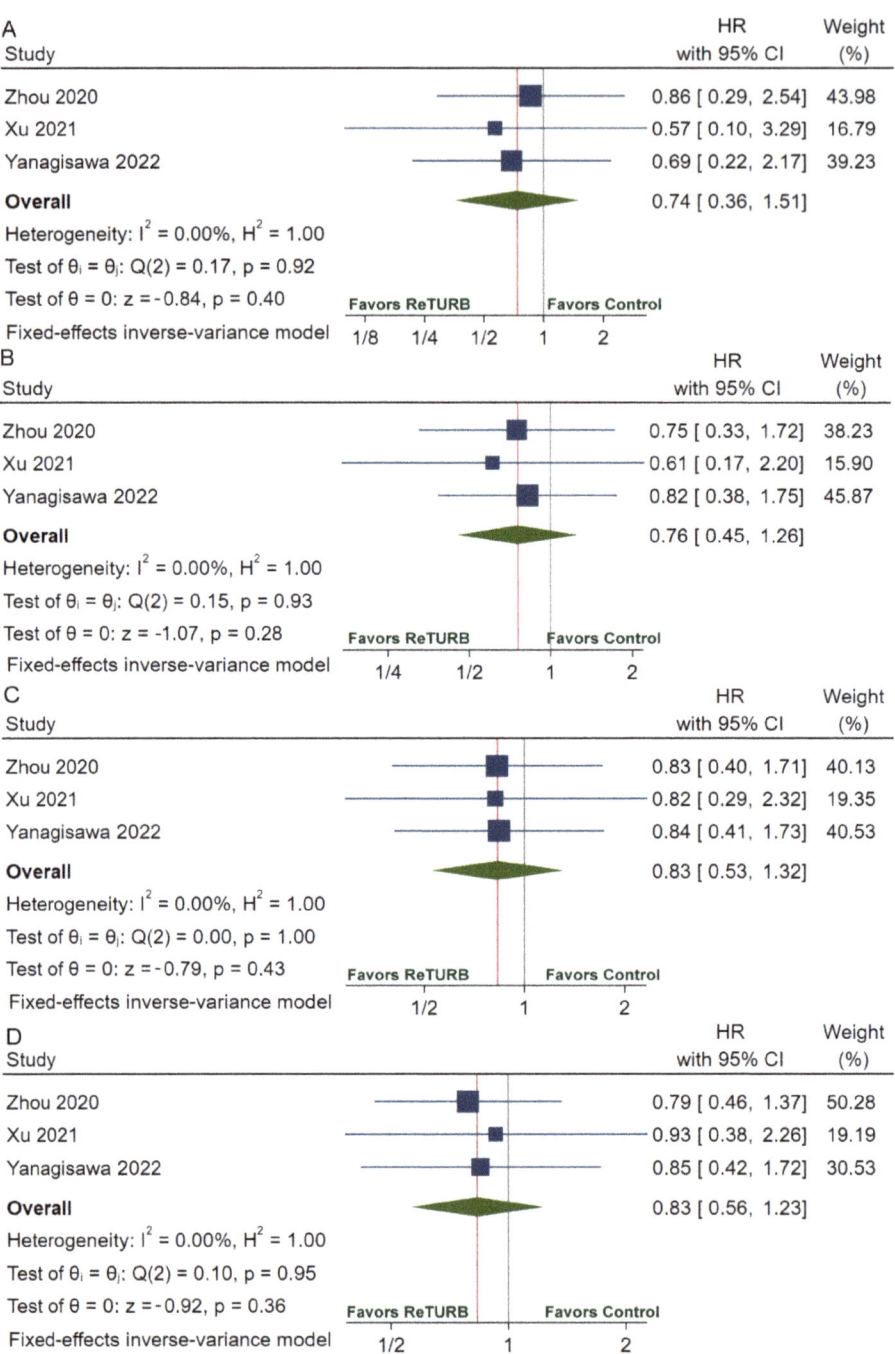

Figure 3. Forests plots of comparisons of 1-year RFS (**A**), 2-year RFS (**B**), 3-year RFS (**C**), and 5-year RFS (**D**) between the reTURB group and control group [32,36,38]. The gray lines represent the reference lines and the red lines show the pooled effect sizes. RFS: recurrence-free survival; HR: hazard ratio; reTURB: repeat transurethral resection of bladder tumors; CI: confidence interval.

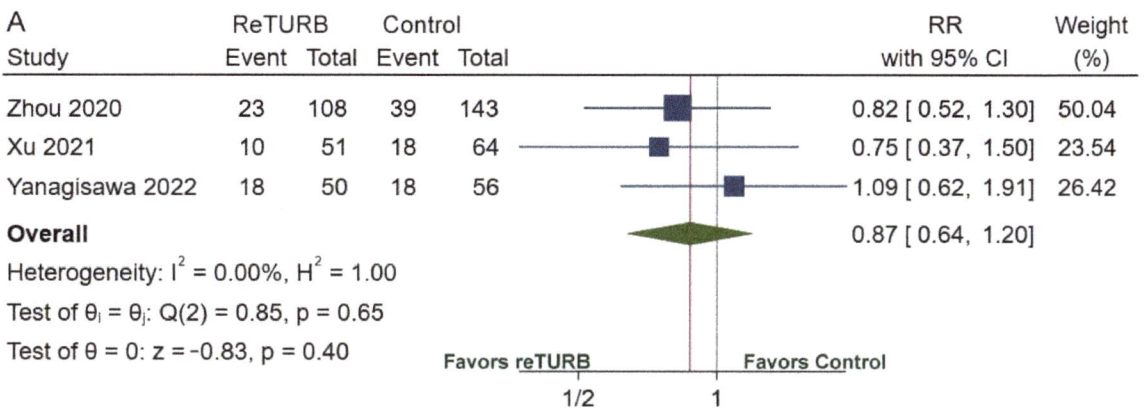
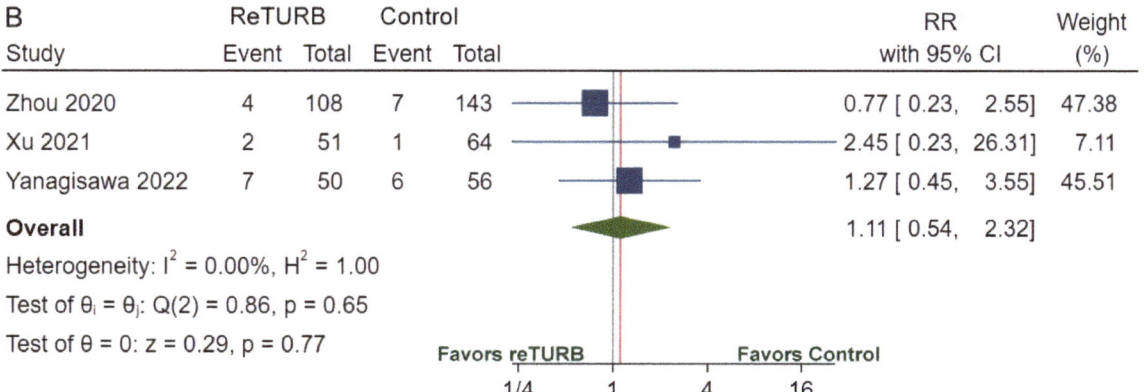

Figure 4. Forests plots of comparisons of recurrence (**A**) and progression (**B**) risk between the reTURB group and control group [32,36,38]. The gray lines represent the reference lines and the red lines show the pooled effect sizes. CI: confidence interval. RR: relative risk; reTURB: repeat transurethral resection of bladder tumors.

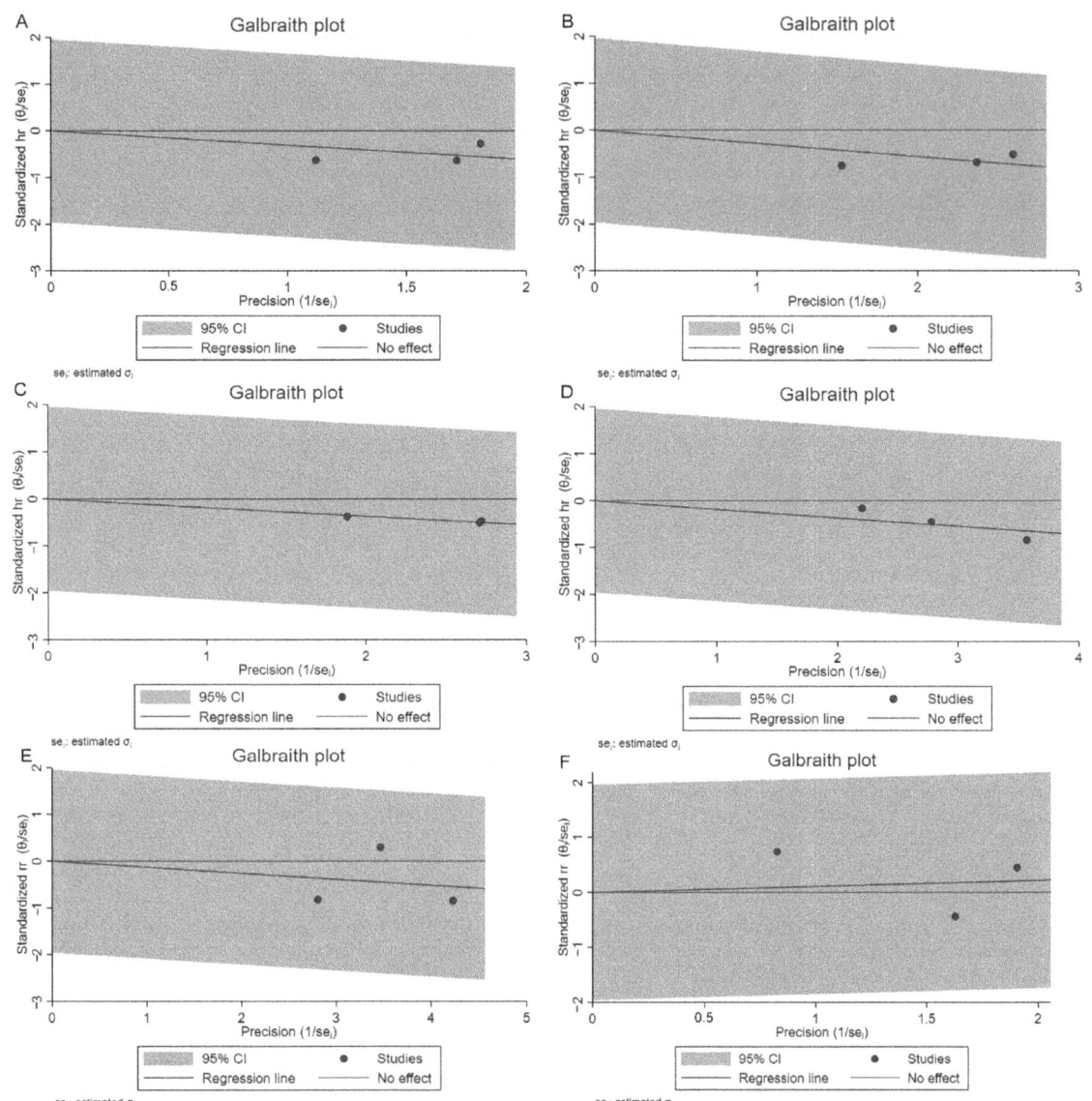

Figure 5. Galbraith plots of comparisons 1-year RFS (**A**), 2-year RFS (**B**), 3-year RFS (**C**), 5-year RFS (**D**), recurrence (**E**) and progression (**F**) between reTURB group and control group. CI: confidence interval.

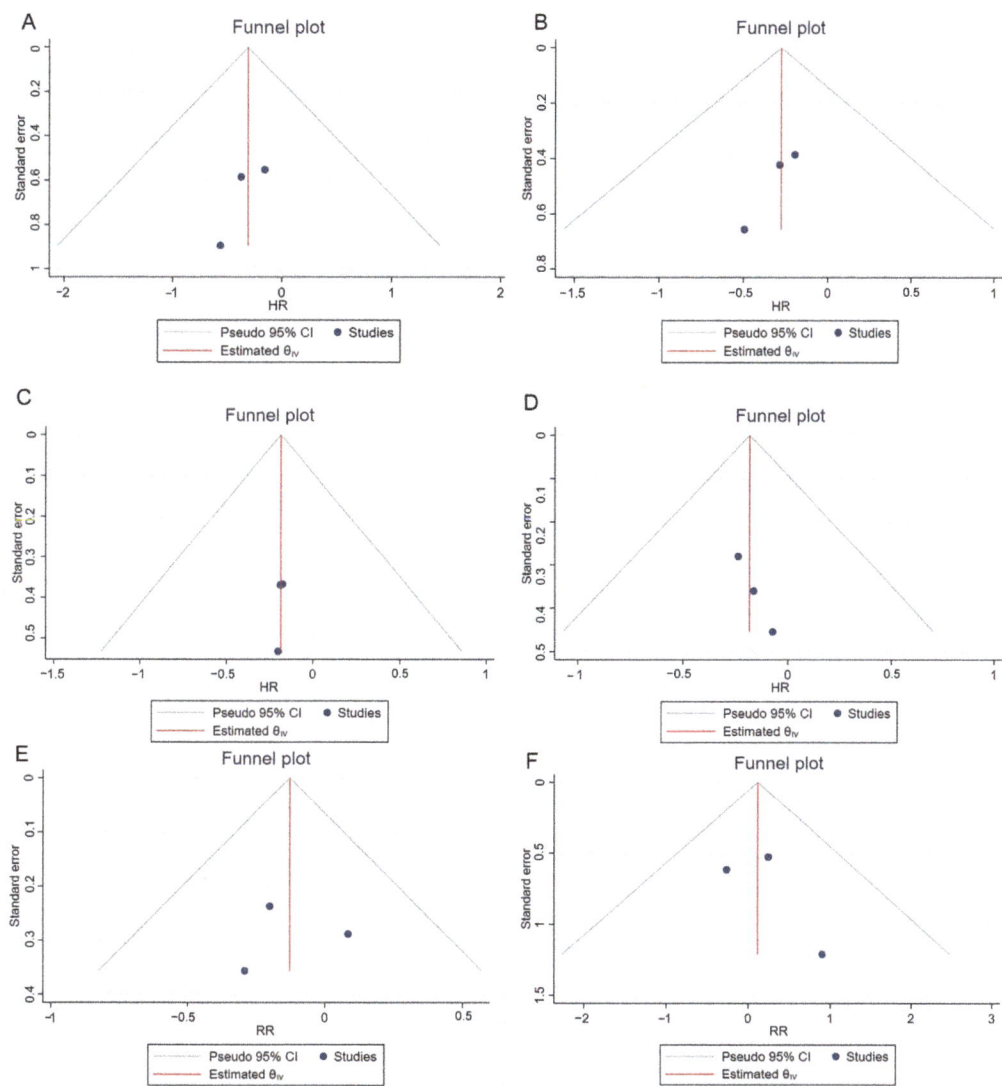

Figure 6. Funnel plots of comparisons 1-year RFS (**A**), 2-year RFS (**B**), 3-year RFS (**C**), 5-year RFS (**D**), recurrence (**E**) and progression (**F**) between reTURB group and control group. CI: confidence interval.

4. Discussion

The cTURB represents the most important endoscopic treatment of bladder tumors. However, cTURB's oncological outcomes have been doubted, given the high residual disease and recurrence rates [4]. For instance, residual tumor at re-resection has been shown in 17–67% of Ta and 20–71% of T1 diseases [39]. Apart from the high incidence of residual and recurrent tumors, cTURB is limited by the risk of understaging due to the absence of DM layer in the specimen, as the presence of DM is a surrogate marker of resection quality which strongly determines prognosis [4,40,41]. An early reTURB is recommended for selected patients to remove any residual disease, restage the tumor and improve the therapeutic outcome. However, most of the previous evidence is based on initial cTURB. Recently, ERBT has emerged as an alternative to cTURB [42]. In contrast to 'piecemeal' resection by cTURB, ERBT incorporates a more delicate en bloc sculpting and tumor excision [43]. ERBT appears safe, feasible, and effective with demonstrably higher rates of DM in the pathologic specimen and provides better staging [6]. Given the excellent quality of the initial resection provided by ERBT and evidence supporting the completeness of tumor resection and reduced residual disease, ERBT might result in less need for reTURB. Therefore, we performed this systematic review to analyze the impact of reTURB on patients who underwent initial ERBT.

A comprehensive review and meta-analysis demonstrate that the residual tumor rate detected by reTURB after ERBT is 5.9% (95%CI, 2.0–11.1%), and the upstaging rate is 0.0% (95%CI, 0.0–0.5%). Residual tumor at reTURB after cTURB has been described in up to 75% of Ta and T1 patients [39]. Even more profound is the rate of upstaging from Ta to T1 or T1 to T2 at reTURB, which has been observed in up to 28% of initial T1 and 9.5% of initial TaHG tumors, respectively [39]. A recent meta-analysis finds that the residual and upstaging rates of T1 BC in reTURB were around 50% and 10%, respectively [44]. All of these are much higher than that of patients who underwent ERBT. If we still do not take the surgical method into account and choose the real "high risk" patients, more patients will take an "unnecessary" reTURB at the risk of perioperative complications and raising the already high cost [45].

In addition, our study shows that RFS was comparable between patients with and without reTURB after initial ERBT. The pooled RRs of recurrence and progression were 0.87 (95%CI, 0.64–1.20; $p = 0.40$) and 1.11 (95%CI, 0.54–2.32; $p = 0.77$), respectively. The two groups have comparable 1-year, 2-year, 3-year, and 5-year RFS. ReTURB seems not to benefit patients who underwent initial ERBT in reducing recurrence and progression. However, a recent meta-analysis demonstrated that short-term RFS (1-year and 3-year) of the reTURB group was better compared with the TURB group. The pooled RR were 1.10 (95%CI: $1.01 \times 10^{1.19}$) and 1.15 (95%CI: 1.03–1.28), respectively [44]. While reTURB did not improve long-term RFS (5-year, 10-year, 15-year) in T1 patients. The pooled RR were 1.12 (95%CI: 0.97–1.30), 1.11 (95%CI: 0.82–1.50) and 1.37 (95%CI: 0.50–3.74), respectively [44]. Nearly all of the included patients had undergone initial cTURB and all the patients with T1 tumors. We cannot do a T1 tumor subgroup analysis as lacking relevant data. But one study included in our review find that the 2-year RFS and 3-year PFS were comparable between patients with T1 tumors who underwent reTURB and those who did not (55.1% vs. 59.9%, $p = 0.6$, 80.6% vs. 82.6%, $p = 0.6$, respectively) [38]. No patient was upstaged to pT2 on reTURB. A reTURB after ERBT for pT1 bladder cancer appears not to improve either recurrence or progression [38].

This study has several limitations. First, the number of included studies and recruited patients in some studies was relatively small. We performed the sensitivity analysis to improve this aspect partially, and the stable results from the sensitivity analysis strengthen our conclusion. There is still no RCT directly investigating the impact of reTURB on the patients receiving ERBT. More studies are urgently needed to clarify this clinical problem further. Second, the baseline characteristics of patients in different studies are not the same, which may influence the prognosis. For example, patients in different studies have different tumor characteristics and follow-up periods. But few studies provided detailed outcomes for subgroup patients, such as patients with Ta or T1 tumors. We were not able to conduct more subgroup analyses to adjust the effect. Although all of these may increase the heterogeneity and confound the results, we find no significant heterogeneity in the statistical test. Third, single-arm studies have an inherent risk of bias. We used the random model to minimize the effect. Because of these limitations, the results of this study should be interpreted with caution.

5. Conclusions

Current evidence demonstrates that reTURB after ERBT for bladder cancer can detect relatively low rates of residual tumor and tumor upstaging and appears not to improve either recurrence or progression. Although the results should be interpreted with caution, our study would assist clinical decisions making when patients who had undergone initial ERBT are informed about the exact effect of reTURB. Further studies are still needed to confirm and clarify the role of reTURB after ERBT.

Supplementary Materials: The following supporting information can be downloaded at: https://www.mdpi.com/article/10.3390/jcm11175049/s1, Table S1. NOS scores of included studies. Table S2. Risk of bias assessment of included studies. Table S3. Egger test and Begg's test for pooled comparisons and sensitivity analysis by trim and fill method. Figure S1. Funnel plots of sensitivity analysis.

Author Contributions: Conceptualization, H.H. and J.Z.; methodology, H.H., M.Z., B.Y. and S.Z.; software, H.H.; validation, M.Z., B.Y. and S.Z.; formal analysis, H.H.; investigation, H.H., M.Z., B.Y., S.Z., Z.L. and J.Z.; data curation, H.H. and J.Z.; writing—original draft preparation, H.H; writing—review and editing, M.Z., B.Y., Z.L. and J.Z.; supervision, Z.L.; funding acquisition, Z.L. All authors have read and agreed to the published version of the manuscript.

Funding: This research was funded by the Natural Science Foundation of Hubei Province (No.ZRMS2020002466); Hubei Chen Xiaoping Science and Technology Development Foundation Youth Science Special Fund (CXPJJH11900018-2010).

Institutional Review Board Statement: Not applicable.

Informed Consent Statement: Not applicable.

Data Availability Statement: Not applicable.

Conflicts of Interest: The authors declare no conflict of interest.

References

1. Richters, A.; Aben, K.K.H.; Kiemeney, L. The global burden of urinary bladder cancer: An update. *World J. Urol.* **2020**, *38*, 1895–1904. [CrossRef] [PubMed]
2. Safiri, S.; Kolahi, A.A.; Naghavi, M.; Global Burden of Disease Bladder Cancer Collaborators. Global, regional and national burden of bladder cancer and its attributable risk factors in 204 countries and territories, 1990–2019: A systematic analysis for the Global Burden of Disease study 2019. *BMJ Glob. Health* **2021**, *6*, e004128. [CrossRef] [PubMed]
3. Babjuk, M.; Burger, M.; Capoun, O.; Cohen, D.; Comperat, E.M.; Dominguez Escrig, J.L.; Gontero, P.; Liedberg, F.; Masson-Lecomte, A.; Mostafid, A.H.; et al. European Association of Urology Guidelines on Non-muscle-invasive Bladder Cancer (Ta, T1, and Carcinoma in Situ). *Eur. Urol.* **2022**, *81*, 75–94. [CrossRef] [PubMed]
4. Kramer, M.W.; Altieri, V.; Hurle, R.; Lusuardi, L.; Merseburger, A.S.; Rassweiler, J.; Struck, J.P.; Herrmann, T.R.W. Current Evidence of Transurethral En-bloc Resection of Nonmuscle Invasive Bladder Cancer. *Eur. Urol. Focus* **2017**, *3*, 567–576. [CrossRef]
5. Ukai, R.; Kawashita, E.; Ikeda, H. A new technique for transurethral resection of superficial bladder tumor in 1 piece. *J. Urol.* **2000**, *163*, 878–879. [CrossRef]
6. Yanagisawa, T.; Mori, K.; Motlagh, R.S.; Kawada, T.; Mostafaei, H.; Quhal, F.; Laukhtina, E.; Rajwa, P.; Aydh, A.; Konig, F.; et al. En Bloc Resection for Bladder Tumors: An Updated Systematic Review and Meta-Analysis of Its Differential Effect on Safety, Recurrence and Histopathology. *J. Urol.* **2022**, *207*, 754–768. [CrossRef]
7. Symeonidis, E.N.; Lo, K.L.; Chui, K.L.; Vakalopoulos, I.; Sountoulides, P. En bloc resection of bladder tumors: Challenges and unmet needs in 2022. *Future Oncol.* **2022**, *18*, 2545–2558. [CrossRef]
8. Teoh, J.Y.; MacLennan, S.; Chan, V.W.; Miki, J.; Lee, H.Y.; Chiong, E.; Lee, L.S.; Wei, Y.; Yuan, Y.; Yu, C.P.; et al. An International Collaborative Consensus Statement on En Bloc Resection of Bladder Tumour Incorporating Two Systematic Reviews, a Two-round Delphi Survey, and a Consensus Meeting. *Eur. Urol.* **2020**, *78*, 546–569. [CrossRef]
9. Powles, T.; Bellmunt, J.; Comperat, E.; De Santis, M.; Huddart, R.; Loriot, Y.; Necchi, A.; Valderrama, B.P.; Ravaud, A.; Shariat, S.F.; et al. Bladder cancer: ESMO Clinical Practice Guideline for diagnosis, treatment and follow-up. *Ann. Oncol.* **2022**, *33*, 244–258. [CrossRef]
10. Chang, S.S.; Boorjian, S.A.; Chou, R.; Clark, P.E.; Daneshmand, S.; Konety, B.R.; Pruthi, R.; Quale, D.Z.; Ritch, C.R.; Seigne, J.D.; et al. Diagnosis and Treatment of Non-Muscle Invasive Bladder Cancer: AUA/SUO Guideline. *J. Urol.* **2016**, *196*, 1021–1029. [CrossRef]
11. Monteiro, L.L.; Witjes, J.A.; Agarwal, P.K.; Anderson, C.B.; Bivalacqua, T.J.; Bochner, B.H.; Boormans, J.L.; Chang, S.S.; Dominguez-Escrig, J.L.; McKiernan, J.M.; et al. ICUD-SIU International Consultation on Bladder Cancer 2017: Management of non-muscle invasive bladder cancer. *World J. Urol.* **2019**, *37*, 51–60. [CrossRef] [PubMed]
12. Bhindi, B.; Kool, R.; Kulkarni, G.S.; Siemens, D.R.; Aprikian, A.G.; Breau, R.H.; Brimo, F.; Fairey, A.; French, C.; Hanna, N.; et al. Canadian Urological Association guideline on the management of non-muscle-invasive bladder cancer—Abridged version. *Can. Urol. Assoc. J.* **2021**, *15*, 230–239. [PubMed]

13. NCC Networks Inc. NCCN Clinical Practice Guidelines in Oncology: Bladder Cancer (Version 2 2022). Available online: https://www.nccn.org/professionals/physician_gls/pdf/bladder.pdf (accessed on 30 June 2022).
14. Huang, J.; Xu, C.; Zhang, X. Chinese Urological Association guidelines on the diagnosis and treatment of bladder cancer. In *Chinese Guidelines on Urological and Andrological Disease*, 2019th ed.; Huang, J., Ed.; China Science Publishing & Media Ltd.: Beijing, China, 2020; pp. 27–84.
15. NICE Guideline: Bladder Cancer: Diagnosis and Management. Available online: https://www.nice.org.uk/guidance/ng2 (accessed on 1 July 2022).
16. Kim, L.H.C.; Patel, M.I. Transurethral resection of bladder tumour (TURBT). *Transl. Androl. Urol.* **2020**, *9*, 3056–3072. [CrossRef]
17. Divrik, R.T.; Sahin, A.F.; Yildirim, U.; Altok, M.; Zorlu, F. Impact of routine second transurethral resection on the long-term outcome of patients with newly diagnosed pT1 urothelial carcinoma with respect to recurrence, progression rate, and disease-specific survival: A prospective randomised clinical trial. *Eur. Urol.* **2010**, *58*, 185–190. [CrossRef]
18. Sfakianos, J.P.; Kim, P.H.; Hakimi, A.A.; Herr, H.W. The effect of restaging transurethral resection on recurrence and progression rates in patients with nonmuscle invasive bladder cancer treated with intravesical bacillus Calmette-Guerin. *J. Urol.* **2014**, *191*, 341–345.
19. Rubio-Briones, J.; Algaba, F.; Gallardo, E.; Marcos-Rodriguez, J.A.; Climent, M.A.; on Behalf of the Sogug Multidisciplinary Working Group. Recent Advances in the Management of Patients with Non-Muscle-Invasive Bladder Cancer Using a Multidisciplinary Approach: Practical Recommendations from the Spanish Oncology Genitourinary (SOGUG) Working Group. *Cancers* **2021**, *13*, 4762. [CrossRef]
20. Del Giudice, F.; Flammia, R.S.; Chung, B.I.; Moschini, M.; Pradere, B.; Mari, A.; Soria, F.; Albisinni, S.; Krajewski, W.; Szydelko, T.; et al. Compared Efficacy of Adjuvant Intravesical BCG-TICE vs. BCG-RIVM for High-Risk Non-Muscle Invasive Bladder Cancer (NMIBC): A Propensity Score Matched Analysis. *Cancers* **2022**, *14*, 887. [CrossRef]
21. Del Giudice, F.; Busetto, G.M.; Gross, M.S.; Maggi, M.; Sciarra, A.; Salciccia, S.; Ferro, M.; Sperduti, I.; Flammia, S.; Canale, V.; et al. Efficacy of three BCG strains (Connaught, TICE and RIVM) with or without secondary resection (re-TUR) for intermediate/high-risk non-muscle-invasive bladder cancers: Results from a retrospective single-institution cohort analysis. *J. Cancer Res. Clin. Oncol.* **2021**, *147*, 3073–3080. [CrossRef]
22. Lee, L.J.; Kwon, C.S.; Forsythe, A.; Mamolo, C.M.; Masters, E.T.; Jacobs, I.A. Humanistic and Economic Burden of Non-Muscle Invasive Bladder Cancer: Results of Two Systematic Literature Reviews. *Clin. Outcomes Res.* **2020**, *12*, 693–709. [CrossRef]
23. Page, M.J.; McKenzie, J.E.; Bossuyt, P.M.; Boutron, I.; Hoffmann, T.C.; Mulrow, C.D.; Shamseer, L.; Tetzlaff, J.M.; Akl, E.A.; Brennan, S.E.; et al. The PRISMA 2020 statement: An updated guideline for reporting systematic reviews. *BMJ* **2021**, *372*, n71. [CrossRef]
24. Wells, G.; Shea, B.; O'Connell, D.; Peterson, J.; Welch, V.; Losos, M.; Tugwell, P. The Newcastle-Ottawa Scale (NOS) for Assessing the Quality of Nonrandomised Studies in Meta-Analyses. Available online: http://www.ohri.ca/programs/clinical_epidemiology/oxford.asp (accessed on 1 June 2022).
25. Knoll, T.; Omar, M.I.; Maclennan, S.; Hernandez, V.; Canfield, S.; Yuan, Y.; Bruins, M.; Marconi, L.; Van Poppel, H.; N'Dow, J.; et al. Key Steps in Conducting Systematic Reviews for Underpinning Clinical Practice Guidelines: Methodology of the European Association of Urology. *Eur. Urol.* **2018**, *73*, 290–300. [CrossRef]
26. Tierney, J.F.; Stewart, L.A.; Ghersi, D.; Burdett, S.; Sydes, M.R. Practical methods for incorporating summary time-to-event data into meta-analysis. *Trials* **2007**, *8*, 16. [CrossRef]
27. Wolters, M.; Kramer, M.W.; Becker, J.U.; Christgen, M.; Nagele, U.; Imkamp, F.; Burchardt, M.; Merseburger, A.S.; Kuczyk, M.A.; Bach, T.; et al. Tm:YAG laser en bloc mucosectomy for accurate staging of primary bladder cancer: Early experience. *World J. Urol.* **2011**, *29*, 429–432. [CrossRef]
28. Muto, G.; Collura, D.; Giacobbe, A.; D'Urso, L.; Muto, G.L.; Demarchi, A.; Coverlizza, S.; Castelli, E. Thulium:yttrium-aluminum-garnet laser for en bloc resection of bladder cancer: Clinical and histopathologic advantages. *Urology* **2014**, *83*, 851–855. [CrossRef]
29. Migliari, R.; Buffardi, A.; Ghabin, H. Thulium laser endoscopic en bloc enucleation of nonmuscle-invasive bladder cancer. *J. Endourol.* **2015**, *29*, 1258–1262. [CrossRef]
30. Hurle, R.; Casale, P.; Lazzeri, M.; Paciotti, M.; Saita, A.; Colombo, P.; Morenghi, E.; Oswald, D.; Colleselli, D.; Mitterberger, M.; et al. En bloc re-resection of high-risk NMIBC after en bloc resection: Results of a multicenter observational study. *World J. Urol.* **2020**, *38*, 703–708. [CrossRef]
31. Yang, Y.; Liu, C.; Yang, X.; Wang, D. Transurethral en bloc resection with monopolar current for non-muscle invasive bladder cancer based on TNM system. *Transl. Cancer Res.* **2020**, *9*, 2210–2219. [CrossRef]
32. Zhou, W.; Wang, W.; Wu, W.; Yan, T.; Du, G.; Liu, H. Can a second resection be avoided after initial thulium laser endoscopic en bloc resection for non-muscle invasive bladder cancer? A retrospective single-center study of 251 patients. *BMC Urol.* **2020**, *20*, 30. [CrossRef]
33. Hashem, A.; Mosbah, A.; El-Tabey, N.A.; Laymon, M.; Ibrahiem, E.-H.; Abd Elhamid, M.; Elshal, A.M. Holmium Laser En-bloc Resection Versus Conventional Transurethral Resection of Bladder Tumors for Treatment of Non-muscle-invasive Bladder Cancer: A Randomized Clinical Trial. *Eur. Urol. Focus* **2021**, *7*, 1035–1043. [CrossRef]
34. Hu, H.; Li, B.; Liu, Z.; Meng, X.; Li, C.; Li, F.; Hu, J.; Chen, Y.; Li, Z.; Wang, S. The individual surgical protocol of transurethral en bloc resection of bladder tumor based on VI-RADS and preliminary experience. *Chin. J. Urol.* **2021**, *42*, 180–184.

35. Poletajew, S.; Krajewski, W.; Stelmach, P.; Adamowicz, J.; Nowak, L.; Moschini, M.; Zapala, P.; Drewa, T.; Paradysz, A.; Radziszewski, P.; et al. En-bloc resection of urinary bladder tumour—A prospective controlled multicentre observational study. *Videosurg. Other Miniinvasive Tech.* **2021**, *16*, 145–150. [CrossRef]
36. Xu, S.; Cao, P.; Wang, K.; Wu, T.; Hu, X.; Chen, H.; Xu, L.; Gu, J.; Wu, S.; Zhu, L.; et al. Clinical Outcomes of Reresection in Patients with High-Risk Nonmuscle-Invasive Bladder Cancer Treated with en Bloc Transurethral Resection: A Retrospective Study with a 1-Year Follow-Up. *J. Endourol.* **2021**, *35*, 1801–1807. [CrossRef]
37. Fan, J.; Zhang, X.; Fan, J.; Li, L.; He, D.; Wu, K. Risk Stratification for the Rate and Location of Residual Bladder Tumor for the Decision of Re-Transurethral Resection of Bladder Tumor. *Front. Oncol.* **2022**, *12*, 788568. [CrossRef]
38. Yanagisawa, T.; Sato, S.; Hayashida, Y.; Okada, Y.; Iwatani, K.; Matsukawa, A.; Kimura, T.; Takahashi, H.; Egawa, S.; Shariat, S.F.; et al. Do we need repeat transurethral resection after en bloc resection for pathological T1 bladder cancer? *BJU Int.* **2022**. [CrossRef]
39. Cumberbatch, M.G.K.; Foerster, B.; Catto, J.W.F.; Kamat, A.M.; Kassouf, W.; Jubber, I.; Shariat, S.F.; Sylvester, R.J.; Gontero, P. Repeat Transurethral Resection in Non-muscle-invasive Bladder Cancer: A Systematic Review. *Eur. Urol.* **2018**, *73*, 925–933. [CrossRef]
40. Soria, F.; Marra, G.; D'Andrea, D.; Gontero, P.; Shariat, S.F. The rational and benefits of the second look transurethral resection of the bladder for T1 high grade bladder cancer. *Transl. Androl. Urol.* **2019**, *8*, 46–53. [CrossRef]
41. Soria, F.; Giordano, A.; Gontero, P. Transurethral resection of bladder tumor and the need for re-transurethral resection of bladder tumor: Time to change our practice? *Curr. Opin. Urol.* **2020**, *30*, 370–376. [CrossRef]
42. Creta, M.; Celentano, G.; Califano, G.; La Rocca, R.; Longo, N. En-bloc Laser Resection of Bladder Tumors: Where Are We Now? *J. Clin. Med.* **2022**, *11*, 3463. [CrossRef]
43. Croghan, S.M.; Compton, N.; Manecksha, R.P.; Cullen, I.M.; Daly, P.J. En bloc transurethral resection of bladder tumors: A review of current techniques. *Can. Urol. Assoc. J.* **2022**, *16*, E287–E293. [CrossRef]
44. Lin, L.; Guo, X.; Ma, Y.; Zhu, J.; Li, X. Does repeat transurethral resection of bladder tumor influence the diagnosis and prognosis of T1 bladder cancer? A systematic review and meta-analysis. *Eur. J. Surg. Oncol.* **2022**. [CrossRef]
45. Wong, V.K.; Ganeshan, D.; Jensen, C.T.; Devine, C.E. Imaging and Management of Bladder Cancer. *Cancers* **2021**, *13*, 1396. [CrossRef] [PubMed]

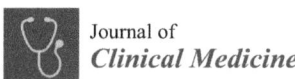

Systematic Review

The Impact of Surgical Waiting Time on Oncological Outcomes in Patients with Upper Tract Urothelial Carcinoma Undergoing Radical Nephroureterectomy: A Systematic Review

Łukasz Nowak [1,*], Wojciech Krajewski [1,*], Jan Łaszkiewicz [1], Bartosz Małkiewicz [1], Joanna Chorbińska [1], Francesco Del Giudice [2], Keiichiro Mori [3], Marco Moschini [4], Krzysztof Kaliszewski [5], Paweł Rajwa [6,7], Ekaterina Laukhtina [6,8], Shahrokh F. Shariat [6,9,10,11,12], Tomasz Szydełko [1] and on behalf of European Association of Urology EAU-Young Academic Urologists YAU Urothelial Cancer Working Party [†]

1. Department of Minimally Invasive and Robotic Urology, University Center of Excellence in Urology, Wroclaw Medical University, 50-556 Wroclaw, Poland; jasieklaszkiewicz@gmail.com (J.Ł.); bmalkiew01@gmail.com (B.M.); joanna.chorbinska@gmail.com (J.C.); tomasz.szydelko1@gmail.com (T.S.)
2. Department of Maternal-Infant and Urological Sciences, Policlinico Umberto I Hospital, "Sapienza" Rome University, 00185 Rome, Italy; francesco.delgiudice@uniroma1.it
3. Department of Urology, The Jikei University School of Medicine, Tokyo 105-8461, Japan; morikeiichiro29@gmail.com
4. Division of Experimental Oncology, Department of Urology, Urological Research Institute, Vita-Salute San Raffaele University, 20132 Milan, Italy; marco.moschini87@gmail.com
5. Department of General, Minimally Invasive and Endocrine Surgery, Wroclaw Medical University, 50-556 Wroclaw, Poland; krzysztof.kaliszewski@umw.edu.pl
6. Department of Urology, Comprehensive Cancer Center, Medical University of Vienna, 1090 Vienna, Austria; pawelgrajwa@gmail.com (P.R.); katyalaukhtina@gmail.com (E.L.); sfshariat@gmail.com (S.F.S.)
7. Department of Urology, Medical University of Silesia, 41-800 Zabrze, Poland
8. Institute for Urology and Reproductive Health, I.M. Sechenov First Moscow State Medical University, 119435 Moscow, Russia
9. Department of Urology, Weill Cornell Medical College, New York, NY 10021, USA
10. Department of Urology, University of Texas Southwestern, Dallas, TX 75390, USA
11. Hourani Center for Applied Scientific Research, Al-Ahliyya Amman University, Amman 19328, Jordan
12. Department of Urology, Second Faculty of Medicine, Charles University, 15006 Prague, Czech Republic
* Correspondence: lllukasz.nowak@gmail.com (Ł.N.); wk@softstar.pl (W.K.); Tel.: +48-717331091 (L.N.); +48-71733101091 (W.K.)
† Members of the European Association of Urology EAU-Young Academic Urologists YAU Urothelial Cancer Working Party listed in the Acknowledgements.

Abstract: Radical nephroureterectomy (RNU) with bladder cuff excision is a standard of care in patients with high-risk upper tract urothelial carcinoma (UTUC). Although several recommendations and guidelines on the delayed treatment of urologic cancers exist, the evidence on UTUC is scarce and ambiguous. The present systematic review aimed to summarize the available evidence on the survival outcomes after deferred RNU in patients with UTUC. A systematic literature search of the three electronic databases (PubMed, Embase, and Cochrane Library) was conducted until 30 April 2022. Studies were found eligible if they reported the oncological outcomes of patients treated with deferred RNU compared to the control group, including those patients treated with RNU without delay. Primary endpoints were cancer-specific survival (CSS), overall survival (OS), and recurrence-free survival (RFS). In total, we identified seven eligible studies enrolling 5639 patients. Significant heterogeneity in the definition of "deferred RNU" was found across the included studies. Three out of five studies reporting CSS showed that deferring RNU was associated with worse CSS. Furthermore, three out of four studies reporting OS found a negative impact of delay in RNU on OS. One out of three studies reporting RFS found a negative influence of delayed RNU on RFS. While most studies reported a 3 month interval as a significant threshold for RNU delay, some subgroup analyses showed that a safe delay for RNU was less than 1 month in patients with ureteral tumors (UT) or less than 2 months in patients with hydronephrosis. In conclusion, long surgical waiting time for RNU (especially more than 3 months after UTUC diagnosis) could be considered as an important risk factor having a negative impact on oncological outcomes in patients with UTUC; however, the results

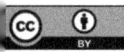

of the particular studies are still inconsistent. The safe delay for RNU might be shorter in specific subsets of high-risk patients, such as those with UT and/or hydronephrosis at the time of diagnosis. High-quality additional studies are required to establish evidence for valid recommendations.

Keywords: upper tract urothelial carcinoma; radical nephroureterectomy; delay; deferred; oncological outcomes

1. Introduction

Upper tract urothelial carcinoma (UTUC) is a rare neoplasm accounting for 5–10% of all urothelial cancers [1]. Radical nephroureterectomy (RNU) with bladder cuff excision is considered to be the treatment of choice in patients with high-risk UTUC, regardless of the primary tumor location [2]. Currently, kidney-sparing surgeries (KSS) are preferred in selected low-risk cases, as they can reduce morbidity without compromising survival endpoints [2].

The issues of surgical prioritization and establishment of recommendations regarding acceptable delays in urological procedures have been of paramount importance for the past months, due to the critical period of the COVID-19 pandemic. Although several valuable recommendations providing an overview of the risks from delayed treatment for urologic cancers exist [3,4], the evidence on UTUC remains scarce and ambiguous.

Apart from limitations of the health care systems and lowered capacity of large-volume centers due to the COVID-19 pandemic [5], multiple other elements can delay RNU. The main patient-related factor influencing the time of RNU is the presence of serious comorbidities that require alignment before surgery, as the vast majority of patients diagnosed with UTUC are elderly [6]. Moreover, some patients can be hesitant to undergo the surgery due to psychological factors. On the other hand, specific disease-related factors, such as administration of neoadjuvant chemotherapy (NAC) or performance of additional diagnostic procedures (e.g., ureteroscopy (URS)), can affect the time of RNU.

The present systematic review aimed to summarize the available evidence on the survival outcomes after deferred RNU in patients with UTUC.

2. Materials and Methods

This systematic review was performed according to the Preferred Reporting Items for Systematic Reviews and Meta-analysis (PRISMA) guidelines and methods outlined in the Cochrane Handbook for Systematic Reviews of Interventions [7,8]. The study protocol was registered a priori on the International Prospective Register of Systematic Reviews (PROSPERO) with the registration number CRD42022303744.

2.1. Search Strategy

A systematic literature search of the three electronic databases (PubMed, Embase, and Cochrane Library) was performed using the following search string: ("upper tract urothelial carcinoma" OR "upper tract urothelial cancer" OR "upper tract urothelial neoplasm" OR "upper urinary tract carcinoma" OR "upper urinary tract cancer" OR "UTUC" OR "UUTC") AND ("nephroureterectomy" OR "RNU" OR "surgery" OR "surgical treatment" OR "operation") AND ("delay" OR "defer" OR "deferred" OR "waiting" OR "time" OR "timing" OR "interval"). The last search was conducted on 30 April 2022. Only articles written in English (without time limitations) were considered. A cross-referenced search was additionally performed from articles selected for full-text review. Moreover, additional articles were screened from ahead-of-print articles published in various urological journals.

2.2. Inclusion and Exclusion Criteria

Studies were assessed for eligibility using the PICO (population, intervention, comparison, outcome) approach. The inclusion criteria were as follows:

- (P)opulation: Patients with UTUC who underwent RNU.
- (I)ntervention: Patients who underwent deferred RNU. Only studies reporting a specific cut-off defining the delay in RNU were included.
- (C)omparison: Patients who underwent RNU without delay.
- (O)utcome: The primary outcomes were cancer-specific survival (CSS) and overall survival (OS). The secondary outcome was recurrence-free survival (RFS).

The general exclusion criteria were as follows: (1) noncomparative studies—reviews, letters, editorial comments, meeting abstracts, replies from authors, case reports; (2) studies not reporting any outcome of interest.

2.3. Data Extraction

Data from eligible studies were independently extracted by two research authors (Ł.N. and J.L.). A standardized data extraction form was created and used to collect: study-related data (first author, publication year, journal, geographical region, study type, study duration, number of patients, reported definition of RNU delay, median time to RNU, follow up period), clinicopathological data (gender, proportion of patients with hydronephrosis, tumor location, RNU approach, pathological tumor stage, pathological tumor grade, proportion of patients with pathologically confirmed lymph node invasion (LNI), proportion of patients with concomitant carcinoma in situ (CIS), proportion of patients with positive lymphovascular invasion (LVI), and proportion of patients who received adjuvant chemotherapy (AC)), and survival data (including 5-year CSS, OS, and RFS rates, as well as their corresponding unadjusted or adjusted hazard ratios (HRs) with 95% confidence intervals (CIs)).

2.4. Quality Assessment and Risk of Bias

The "risk of bias" (RoB) for the selected studies was independently assessed by two review authors (Ł.N. and W.K.) according to the principles outlined in the Cochrane Handbook for Systematic Reviews and Interventions [8]. The articles were assessed in terms of allocation, sequence generation and concealment, blinding of participants, personnel and outcome assessors, completeness of outcome data, selective outcome reporting, and other sources of bias. The selected studies were also reviewed based on the adjustment for the effect of the following confounders: pathological tumor stage, pathological tumor grade, concomitant CIS, LVI, LNI, and tumor location. The risk of confounding bias was considered to be high if the confounder was not controlled for in multivariate analysis.

3. Results

3.1. Literature Search Results

The PRISMA flow chart summarizing the process of study selection was presented in Figure 1. The initial literature search identified 1258 potentially relevant references. Using literature manager software—Endnote 20 (Clarivate)—346 duplicate records were removed. After screening the titles and abstracts of identified papers, 487 and 20 articles were excluded, due to inappropriate type (e.g., review, case series, meeting abstract) and non-English language, respectively. Among the remaining 405 original studies, 389 were not relevant to the present systematic review, leaving 16 potentially eligible papers. Of the 16 full-text articles assessed for eligibility, 9 were excluded based on the predefined selection criteria.

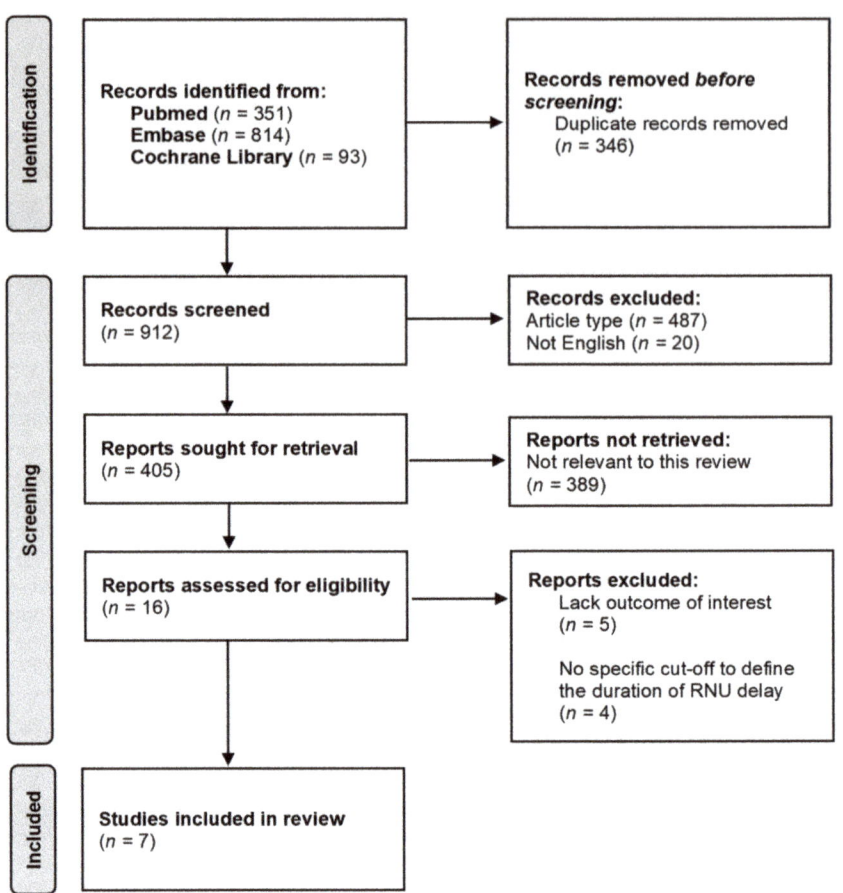

Figure 1. A PRISMA flowchart describing the study selection process. RNU = radical nephroureterectomy.

3.2. Features of Included Studies

Finally, we included seven full-text studies (Table 1) [9–15]. Overall, the included studies enrolled 5639 patients. All articles were retrospective series, of which: three were single-center series [10,12,15], three were multi-center series [9,11,13], and one was population-based registry (data from the National Cancer Database, NCDB) [14]. One study provided data from a worldwide dataset [13], while the remaining papers included data from Asian (n = 3) [9,10,15], North American (n = 2) [12,14], and European (n = 1) [11] populations.

The clinical and pathological characteristics of cohorts were provided in Table 2. Most of the patients were male (54.8%) [10–15]. The proportion of non-muscle-invasive (<pT2) and muscle-invasive tumors (≥pT2) was roughly equal in four articles [11–14], while another three studies reported a higher proportion of muscle-invasive tumors [9,10,15]. Predominance of grade 3 (G3) or high-grade (HG) tumors was observed in all included studies. LNI and LVI rates ranged from 4.1% to 12.5% and 12% to 30.8%, respectively. The proportion of patients receiving AC ranged from 10 to 31.2%. All studies except one [12] excluded patients who received NAC before RNU.

Table 1. Baseline characteristics of included studies.

First Author, Year [Reference]	Journal	Geographical Region	Study Type	Study Duration	Number of Patients	Definition of RNU Delay	Median Time to RNU, Days	Follow up, Months	Reported Outcomes
Lee H.Y. et al., 2021 [9]	Urologic Oncology: Seminars and Original Investigations	Asia	Retrospective Multi-center	2000–2019	665	Group 1: ≤90 days Group 2: >90 days	NR	Group 1: mean 52.3 Group 2: mean 34.2	OS
Lee J.N. et al., 2014 [10]	Journal of Surgical Oncology	Asia	Retrospective Single-center	2001–2010	138	Group 1: ≤30 days Group 2: >30 days	Mean: 16.6 Mean: 70.1	All patients: median 40	CSS, RFS
Nison et al., 2013 [11]	World Journal of Urology	Europe	Retrospective Multi-center	1995–2011	512	Group 1: ≤30 days Group 2: 31–60 days Group 3: 61–90 days Group 4: >90 days	NR	All patients: median 23.6	CSS, RFS
Sundi et al., 2013 [12]	Urologic Oncology	North America	Retrospective Single-center	1990–2007	240	Group 1: ≤90 days Group 2: >90 days	Mean: 24 Mean: 432	All patients: median 29	CSS, OS
Waldert et al., 2009 [13]	BJU International	Multinational	Retrospective Multi-center	2000–2007	187	Group 1: ≤90 days Group 2: >90 days	Median: 33 Median: 110	All patients: median 47.5	CSS, RFS
Xia et al., 2017 [14]	Urologic Oncology: Seminars and Original Investigations	North America	Retrospective Population-based registry	2004–2013	3581	Group 1: 8–30 days Group 2: 1–7 days Group 3: 31–60 days Group 4: 61–90 days Group 5: 91–120 days Group 6: 121–180 days	NR	All patients: median 40.4	OS
Zhao et al., 2021 [15]	Frontiers in Oncology	Asia	Retrospective Single-center	2008–2019	316	Group 1: ≤30 days Group 2: 31–90 days Group 3: >90 days	Median: 12 Median: 42 Median: 191	All patients: median 43	OS, CSS

Abbreviations: CSS = cancer-specific survival; NR = not reported; OS = overall survival; RFS = recurrence-free survival; RNU = radical nephroureterectomy.

Table 2. Clinical and pathological characteristics of main cohorts in included studies.

First Author, Year [Reference]	Gender, n (%)	Preoperative Hydronephrosis, n (%)	URS, n (%)	Tumor Location, n (%)	RNU Approach, n (%)	Pathological Tumor stage, n (%)	Pathological Tumor grade, n (%)	LNI, n (%)	Concomitant CIS, n (%)	LVI, n (%)	AC, n (%)
Lee H.Y. et al., 2021 [9]	Male: 297 (49.5) Female: 303 (50.5)	NR	Yes: 491 (74.0) No: 174 (26.0)	NR	NR	<T2: 198 (33.0) ≥T2: 361 (67.0)	G1: 77 (14.8) G2: 62 (11.9) G3: 381 (73.3)	Yes: 44 (7.3) No ª: 556 (92.7)	Yes: 20 (3.3) No: 580 (96.7)	Yes: 133 (22.2) No: 467 (77.8)	Yes: 89 (14.8) No: 511 (85.2)
Lee J.N. et al., 2014 [10]	Male: 96 (69.6) Female: 42 (30.4)	Yes: 100 (72.5) No: 38 (27.5)	NR	RPT: 58 (42.0) UT: 80 (58.0)	Open: 36 (26.1) Laparoscopic: 102 (73.9)	<T2: 50 (36.2) ≥T2: 88 (63.8)	LG: 46 (33.3) HG: 92 (66.7)	Yes: 10 (7.2) No ª: 128 (92.8)	Yes: 7 (5.1) No: 131 (94.9)	Yes: 27 (19.6) No: 111 (80.4)	Yes: 43 (31.2) No: 95 (68.8)
Nison et al., 2013 [11]	Male: 348 (68.0) Female: 164 (32.0)	NR	Yes: 170 (33.2) No: 342 (66.8)	RPT: 277 (54.1) UT: 172 (33.6) Multifocal: 63 (12.3)	NR	<T2: 252 (49.2) ≥T2: 260 (50.8)	G1: 62 (12.1) G2: 154 (30.1) G3: 296 (57.8)	Yes: 39 (7.6) No ª: 473 (92.4)	NR	Yes: 126 (24.6) No: 368 (75.4)	NR
Sundi et al., 2013 [12]	Male: 157 (65.4) Female: 83 (34.6)	NR	NR	RPT: 140 (58.3) UT: 100 (41.7)	NR	<T2: 120 (50.0) ≥T2: 120 (50.0)	LG: 51 (21.2) HG: 189 (78.8)	Yes: 30 (12.5) No ª: 210 (87.5)	Yes: 101 (42.1) No: 139 (57.9)	Yes: 74 (30.8) No: 166 (69.2)	Yes: 38 (15.8) No: 202 (84.2)
Waldert et al., 2009 [13]	Male: 150 (80.2) Female: 37 (19.8)	NR	Yes: 49 (26.2) No: 138 (73.8)	RPT: 88 (47.1) UT: 99 (52.9)	Open: 151 (80.7) Laparoscopic: 36 (19.3)	<T2: 97 (51.9) ≥T2: 90 (48.1)	LG: 62 (33.2) HG: 125 (66.8)	Yes: 17 (9.1) No ª: 170 (90.9)	Yes: 78 (41.7) No: 109 (58.3)	Yes: 54 (28.9) No: 133 (71.1)	Yes: 30 (16.0) No: 157 (84.0)
Xia et al., 2017 [14]	Male: 2038 (56.9) Female: 1543 (43.1)	NR	NR	RPT: 2428 (67.8) UT: 1153 (32.2)	NR	<T2: 1865 (52.1) ≥T2: 1429 (41.7)	G1-2: 1273 (35.6) G3-4: 2308 (64.4)	Yes: 147 (4.1) No ª: 3434 (95.9)	NR	NR	Yes: 357 (10.0) No: 3224 (90.0)
Zhao et al., 2021 [15]	Male: 205 (64.9) Female: 111 (35.1)	Yes: 158 (50.0) No: 158 (50.0)	NR	RPT: 173 (54.7) UT: 143 (45.3)	Open: 67 (21.2) Laparoscopic: 249 (78.8)	<T2: 87 (27.5) ≥T2: 229 (72.5)	LG: 81 (25.6) HG: 234 (74.4)	Yes: 34 (10.8) No ª: 282 (89.2)	NR	Yes: 38 (12.0) No: 278 (88.0)	Yes: 32 (10.1) No: 284 (89.9)

ª pathological N0 and/or Nx. Abbreviations: AC = adjuvant chemotherapy; CIS = carcinoma in situ; HG = high grade; LG = low grade; LNI = lymph node invasion; LVI = lymphovascular invasion; NR = not reported; RNU = radical nephroureterectomy; RPT = renal pelvic tumor; URS = ureteroscopy; UT = ureteral tumor.

Several publications provided additional analyses of specific subset of patients extracted from the main cohorts. Lee J.K. et al. stratified patients by primary tumor location (separate analyses for renal pelvic tumors (RPT) and ureteral tumors (UT)) [10]. Zhao et al. conducted additional analyses for patients stratified by the presence of hydronephrosis at the time of diagnosis [15]. Sundi et al. provided separate outcome analysis for patients who did not receive NAC [12]. Waldert et al. and Xia et al. separately analyzed a muscle-invasive cohort (patients with ≥pT2 tumors) or a "higher-risk" cohort (patients with ≥pT2 and/or ≥G3 tumors), respectively [13,14].

Only two studies reported the reasons for RNU delay. In Sundi et al.'s study, 50% of delayed RNU were caused by an administration of NAC, while an additional 17% were delayed because of the initial endoscopic management [12]. Performance of URS before RNU was the main cause of delay in the study by Nison et al. [11].

3.3. Risk of Bias (RoB) and Quality Assessment of Included Studies

The evaluation of RoB and confounding assessment for included studies is shown in Figure 2. Due to the retrospective design, all selected articles carried a high RoB. The issue of confounding was addressed by most studies, as statistical adjustment was performed in five out of seven articles through multivariate analyses [9,10,12,14,15]. Of them, all were adjusted for pathological tumor stage and grade. However, other confounders were not uniformly taken into account.

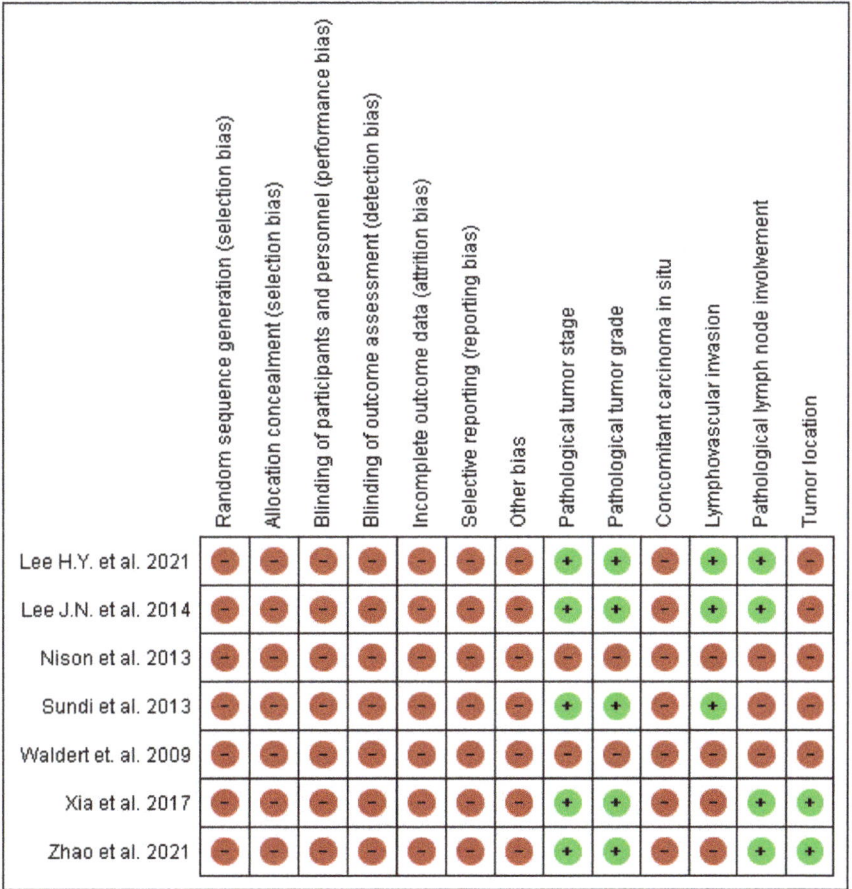

Figure 2. The risk of bias and confounding assessment for included studies [9–15].

3.4. Definition of Deferred Radical Nephroureterectomy

Surgical wait time was predominantly defined as the interval between initial imaging diagnosis and radical surgery of UTUC. Significant heterogeneity in the definition of "deferred RNU" was found across the included studies. Three reports (Lee H.Y. et al., Sundi et al., Waldert et al.) used a cut-off of 90 days (3 months) [9,12,13], while a single study (Lee J.N. et al.) used a cut-off of 30.5 days (1 month) [10]. Nison et al. used the following delay intervals: ≤30 days (<1 month), 31–60 days (1–2 months), 61–90 days (2–3 months), >90 days (>3 months) [11]. Zhao et al. presented groups categorized by the following time intervals: ≤30 days (<1 month), 31–90 days (1–3 months), >90 days (>3 months) [15]. Xia et al. divided patients into those who underwent RNU: 1–7 days, 8–30 days, 31–60 days (1–2 months), 61–90 days (2–3 month), 91–120 days (3–4 months), and 121–180 days (4–6 months) after UTUC diagnosis [14].

3.5. Results of Systematic Review (Qualitative Synthesis)

3.5.1. Cancer-Specific Survival (CSS)

Data regarding CSS were reported in five out of seven studies (Table 3) [9,10,12,13,15]. Of them, three found a significant impact of the delay in RNU on CSS in the overall cohort or a subset of patients [10,13,15].

Lee J.N. et al. observed no significant difference in CSS between patients who underwent RNU ≤ 30 days or >30 days after UTUC diagnosis [10]. However, subgroup analysis of patients with UT revealed that CSS was significantly improved in patients who had RNU within 30 days (5-year CSS: 87.9% vs. 54.5%, $p < 0.001$). Multivariable Cox regression analysis confirmed that a surgical wait time of more than 1 month was one of the independent prognostic factors of worse CSS in a subset of patients with UT (HR = 6.26, 95% CI: 1.90–20.62, $p = 0.003$). However, no association was found in a subset of patients with RPT [10]. Using univariable Cox regression analysis, Nison et al. found no significant differences in CSS for any reported time interval, even in a subset of patients with confirmed muscle-invasive UTUC [11]. Sundi et al. demonstrated no significant differences between the "early" (≤90 days) and "delayed" (>90 days) RNU groups with respect to 5-year CSS rates in the overall cohort (71.6% vs. 70.6%, $p > 0.05$), as well as in a subset of patients who did not receive NAC (71.6% vs. 81.5%, $p > 0.05$) [12]. Waldert et al. showed no significant difference in CSS between patients who had RNU at ≤ 90 days or > 90 days after UTUC diagnosis (5-year CSS: 72% vs. 63%, $p = 0.153$) [13]. In univariate Cox regression analysis, the time from diagnosis to RNU (as a continuous variable) was associated with worse CSS in a subset of patients with muscle-invasive disease (HR = 1.005, 95% CI: 1.001–1.010, $p = 0.003$); this was not true for the whole cohort ($p = 0.658$) [13]. Zhao et al. noted no significant difference in CSS for patients undergoing RNU at 31–90 days compared with ≤30 days; however, those with a delay > 90 days had a significantly worse CSS (65.8% vs. 70.9% vs. 39.6%, $p = 0.032$) [15]. In multivariate Cox regression analysis, performed for a subset of patients with hydronephrosis at the time of UTUC diagnosis, surgical wait time > 60 days was one of the independent risk factors for worse CSS (HR = 1.74, 95% CI: 1.07–2.82, $p = 0.026$) [15].

The initially planned meta-analysis for CSS was not possible because of the paucity and heterogeneity of available data.

Table 3. Primary oncological outcomes of interest reported in included studies.

First Author, Year [Reference]	Subgroup	5-Year CSS	p-Value	5-Year OS	p-Value	Multivariable Cox Regression Analysis—CSS HR [95% CI]	p-Value	Multivariable Cox Regression Analysis—OS HR [95% CI]	p-Value
Lee H.Y. et al., 2021 [9]	NA	NR	NR	Delay ≤ 90 days: 72.9% Delay > 90 days: 63.5%	0.015 *	NR	NR	Delay ≤ 90 days: Ref Delay > 90 days: 1.55 [1.03–2.33]	0.035 *
Lee J.N. et al., 2014 [10]	All patients	Delay ≤ 30 days: 77.3% Delay > 30 days: 69.1%	0.087	NR	NR	NR	Univariable 0.089	NR	NR
	Renal pelvis tumors	Delay ≤ 30 days: 63.9% Delay > 30 days: 90.1%	0.084	NR	NR	NR	Univariable 0.085	NR	NR
	Ureteral tumors	Delay ≤ 30 days: 87.9% Delay > 30 days: 54.5%	<0.001 *	NR	NR	Delay ≤ 30 days: ref Delay > 30 days: 6.26 [1.90–20.62]	0.003 *	NR	NR
Nison et al., 2013 [11]	NA	NR	NR	NR	NR	Univariable Delay ≤ 30 days: ref Delay 31–60 days: 1.00 [0.50–1.98] Delay 61–90 days: 0.84 [0.37–1.91] Delay > 90 days: 0.92 [0.45–1.89]	0.99 0.68 0.68	NR	NR
Sundi et al., 2013 [12]	All patients	Delay ≤ 90 days: 71.6% Delay > 90 days: 70.6%	NS	Delay ≤ 90 days: 61.3% Delay > 90 days: 77.0%	NS	NR	NR	Delay ≤ 90 days: ref Delay > 90 days: 1.54 [0.73–3.25]	0.25
	Patients not receiving NAC	Delay ≤ 90 days: 71.6% Delay > 90 days: 81.5%	NS	Delay ≤ 90 days: 61.3% Delay > 90 days: 77%	NS	NR	NR	Delay ≤ 90 days: ref Delay > 90 days: 0.94 [0.28–3.08]	0.92
Waldert et al., 2009 [13]	All patients	Delay ≤ 90 days: 72% Delay > 90 days: 63%	NS	NR	NR	Univariable Time as continuous variable: 1.00 [0.99–1.01]	0.658	NR	NR
	≥pT2 on RNU	Delay ≤ 90 days: 49% Delay > 90 days: 45%	NS	NR	NR	Time as continuous variable: 1.005 [1.001–1.010]	0.03	NR	NR
Xia et al., 2017 [14]	All patients	NR	NR	Delay 8–30 days: 64.2% Delay 1–7 days: 58.5% Delay 31–60 days: 61.8% Delay 61–90 days: 60.6% Delay 91–120 days: 61.5% Delay 121–180 days: 36.6%	*	NR	NR	Delay 8–30 days: ref Delay 1–7 days: 1.32 [1.06–1.67] Delay 31–60 days: 1.11 [0.97–1.27] Delay 61–90 days: 1.09 [0.91–1.30] Delay 91–120 days: 1.00 [0.74–1.35] Delay 121–180 days: 1.61 [1.19–2.19]	– 0.016 * 0.126 0.360 0.976 0.002 *
	≥pT2 and/or ≥G3 on RNU	NR	NR	Delay 8–30 days: 57.2% Delay 1–7 days: 55.8% Delay 31–60 days: 53.5% Delay 61–90 days: 51.6% Delay 91–120 days: 51.6% Delay 121–180 days: 26.5%	*	NR	NR	Delay 8–30 days: ref Delay 1–7 days: 1.24 [0.95–1.61] Delay 31–60 days: 1.10 [0.94–1.27] Delay 61–90 days: 1.07 [0.88–1.31] Delay 91–120 days: 0.94 [0.66–1.34] Delay 121–180 days: 1.56 [1.11–2.20]	– 0.114 0.231 0.510 0.744 0.010 *
Zhao et al., 2021 [15]	All patients	Delay ≤ 30 days: 65.8% Delay 31–90 days: 70.9% Delay > 90 days: 39.6%	0.032 *	Delay ≤ 30 days: 56.4% Delay 31–90 days: 59.3% Delay > 90 days: 35.1%	0.045 *	NR	NR	NR	NR
	Patients with hydronephrosis	Delay ≤ 60 days: 61.7% Delay > 60 days: 49.1%	0.041 *	Delay ≤ 60 days: 55.1% Delay > 60 days: 44.2%	0.023 *	Delay ≤ 60 days: ref Delay > 60 days: 1.74 [1.07–2.82]	0.026 *	Delay ≤ 60 days: ref Delay > 60 days: 2.05 [1.20–3.50]	0.009 *

* Statistically significant p-value. Abbreviations: CI = confidence interval; CSS = cancer-specific survival; HR = hazard ratio; OS = overall survival; NA = not applicable; NR = not reported; NS = not statistically significant; RNU = radical nephroureterectomy.

3.5.2. Overall Survival (OS)

Data regarding OS were reported in four out of seven studies (Table 3) [9,12,14,15]. Three of them found a significant impact of delay in RNU on OS in the overall cohort or a subset of patients [9,14,15].

Lee H.Y. et al. showed that an "early" ($\leq$90 days) RNU group had a better 5-year OS rate, compared to a "delayed" (>90 days) RNU group (72.9% vs. 63.5%, p = 0.015) [9]. In addition, on multivariate Cox regression analysis, RNU after 90 days was associated with a significantly worse OS (HR = 1.55, 95% CI: 1.03–2.33, p = 0.035) [9]. Conversely, Sundi et al. found no significant difference in OS between patients undergoing RNU at $\leq$90 days and >90 days from UTUC diagnosis [12]. Xia et al. demonstrated that patients with RNU delay time of 31–60 days, 61–90 days, and 91–120 days had similar OS compared with patients who had a delay in RNU of 8—30 days in both the overall cohort and "higher-risk" cohort ($\geq$pT2 and/or $\geq$G3 tumors) [14]. However, patients with RNU deferred for 121–180 days had worse OS in both overall (HR = 1.61, 95% CI: 1.19–2.19, p = 0.002) and "higher-risk" ($\geq$pT2 and/or $\geq$G3 tumors; HR = 1.56, 95% CI: 1.11–2.20, p = 0.01) cohorts, respectively [14]. Zhao et al. showed no significant difference in OS for patients undergoing RNU at 31–90 days, compared with $\leq$30 days. However, those with a delay >90 days had worse OS (56.4% vs. 59.3% vs. 35.1%, p = 0.045) [15]. On multivariate Cox regression analysis of patients with hydronephrosis at the time of diagnosis, surgical wait time > 60 days was one of the independent risk factors for worse OS (HR = 2.05, 95% CI: 1.20–3.50, p = 0.009) [15].

A forest plot comparing OS between "long" and "short" surgical waiting time groups is provided in Supplementary Figure S1.

3.5.3. Recurrence-Free Survival (RFS)

Data regarding RFS were reported in three out of seven studies [10,11,13]. Of them, one found a significant impact of the delay in RNU on RFS in the overall cohort or a subset of patients [10].

Five-year RFS rates reported by Lee J.N. et al. were comparable between patients who underwent RNU $\leq$ 30 days or >30 days after UTUC diagnosis (77.6% vs. 73.9%, p = 0.534) [10]. In a subset of patients with RPT, delay in RNU > 30 days was associated with improved 5-year RFS rate (66.3% vs. 91.6%, p = 0.028). However, it was not confirmed in the univariable Cox regression analysis (p = 0.537). In a subgroup analysis including patients with UT, the delay in RNU > 30 days was associated with significantly worse 5-year RFS (85.6% vs. 60.7%, p = 0.007) and was one of the independent prognostic factors for worse RFS in multivariable Cox regression analysis (HR = 4.120, 95% CI: 1.38–12.30, p = 0.011) [10]. Nison et al. found no significant difference in RFS for any reported time interval (delay < 1 month as a reference, delay > 3 months: HR = 0.96, 95% CI: 0.70–1.29, p = 0.78) [11]. Furthermore, in another study from Waldert et al., patients who underwent RNU > 90 days after UTUC diagnosis had similar 5-year RFS compared to those who underwent RNU $\leq$ 90 days (68% vs. 51%, p = 0.066) [13].

The initially planned meta-analysis for RFS was not possible because of the paucity and heterogeneity of available data.

4. Discussion

In the present systematic review, we conducted a qualitative synthesis of current data regarding the impact of delaying RNU on long-term oncological outcomes in patients with UTUC. According to the current evidence, long surgical waiting time for RNU (especially beyond 3 months after UTUC diagnosis) could be considered as an important risk factor having a negative impact on survival parameters. Notably, the "safe window" for RNU seems to be shorter specifically for high-risk patients such as those diagnosed with UT or hydronephrosis.

Diagnosis of UTUC and proper preoperative determination of the disease stage and grade can often be challenging. As it is a crucial step in terms of planning the treatment (conservative management vs. RNU), diagnostic URS with biopsy is a valuable tool in case of inconclusive computed tomography urography (CTU) findings. Even though URS may clearly increase the time between diagnosis and treatment, it is rarely associated with a long delay (e.g., more than 3 months). In a single study included in the present systematic review, patients who underwent URS and delayed RNU had similar CSS and RFS compared to the patients who underwent RNU without previous URS [11]. Nonetheless, the results of a recent meta-analysis including 16 retrospective series confirmed that URS with biopsy followed by RNU could be associated with significantly worse intravesical RFS (but not with CSS, OS, and metastasis-free-survival), compared to RNU alone [16]. These findings could be explained by increased risk of tumor seeding during endoscopic biopsy or the manipulation of the ureteroscope. Therefore, URS (particularly with biopsy) seems reasonable only in uncertain diagnostic cases, when no NAC is planned and the disease cannot be classified as high-risk based on other clinical factors, such as tumor size, multifocality (based on CTU results) or high-grade cytology results.

Currently, KSS (e.g., endoscopic ablation, segmental ureteral resection) is the preferred approach in low-risk UTUC. Gadzinski et al. showed that the delay in RNU related to previous KSS did not affect survival outcomes in patients with UTUC [17]. No specific cut-off for delay interval was reported and the study included a relatively small sample size (n = 73). Authors reported comparable 5-year OS (64% vs. 59%) and 5-year CSS (91% vs. 80%) between patients in the delayed RNU group (with previous conservative treatment) and immediate RNU group (without previous conservative treatment). However, a significant pathologic progression was observed in 43% of the cases in the delayed surgical group, when compared to the initial endoscopic pathology. In another multi-institutional retrospective study, Gurbuz et al. confirmed that endoscopic ablation prior to RNU was not associated with decreased CSS and disease-free survival (DFS) [18]. This evidence suggests that delayed RNU preceded by KSS could be a feasible option after endoscopic management failure; however, proper patient selection for initial KSS seems to be the key to guaranteeing satisfactory oncological outcomes [17,18].

Ureteral location is considered as an important negative prognostic factor in patients with UTUC. Recent meta-analysis including 10,537 patients with RPT and 6299 patients with UT demonstrated that ureteral location of UTUC is associated with decreased CSS, OS, and DFS [19]. More aggressive behavior of UT, potentially related to tumor's surrounding environment (e.g., thin periureteral layer of muscular and fatty tissue, compared to renal parenchyma), raises the question about the safe delay interval in radical treatment. Based on the results of Lee et al.'s study, a surgical wait time of more than 1 month after UTUC diagnosis might be associated with significantly worse prognosis in patients with UT [10]. In addition, a shorter "safe window" for radical treatment was noted by Zhao et al. for patients with UTUC presenting hydronephrosis at the time of diagnosis [15]. In this cohort, the CSS and OS of the patients with surgical wait time of more than 60 days were significantly lower than those of patients with surgical wait time of less than 60 days. To support their results, the authors hypothesized that increased pressure of the renal pelvis and ureter due to hydronephrosis may lead to easier peripheral invasion or ischemic changes in surrounding tissues, inducing the expression of hypoxia-inducible factors involved in tumor growth [15]. Moreover, a variety of independent factors can influence oncological outcomes, regardless of surgical waiting time. Pathological stage, grade, LNI, LVI, positive surgical margin, presence of tumor necrosis, hydronephrosis, and tumor size were also associated with worse CSS and OS in several selected studies [10–12,15]. OS was negatively influenced by pathological tumor grade, stage, size, multifocality, LNI and hydronephrosis [9,15]. Therefore, surgical waiting time should not be considered as the sole independent risk factor of worse oncological outcomes in patients with UTUC. In view of the abovementioned evidence, determining the safe delay of the RNU should be conducted according to the individual case risk profile, based on all available clinical factors. Nevertheless, further studies are required to make strict recommendations.

It needs to be emphasized that the delay in RNU does not always delay the treatment. There is growing evidence that cisplatin-based NAC can lead to a significant downstaging or a complete response on final pathologic examination of the RNU specimen (resulting in CSS and OS improvement), which is why NAC is increasingly utilized in the management of UTUC [20]. On the other hand, NAC might delay surgical treatment of UTUC, potentially leading to disease progression in chemo-resistant patients [21]. In addition, patients undergoing NAC may suffer from toxicities related to chemotherapy, which may delay surgery even further [21]. Thus, development and validation of preoperative models are extremely important as the scope of future research, in order to guide selection of the most suitable patients with UTUC who will benefit from NAC. Unfortunately, selected papers did not include subgroup analyses of patients receiving NAC before RNU. [11]. Only one study by Sundi et al. addressed this issue and demonstrated no significant differences in CSS between the "early" ($\leq$90 days) and "delayed" (>90 days) RNU groups in a total cohort (50% of patients receiving NAC) and subgroup of patients not receiving NAC. Therefore, due to paucity of data, the safe delay in RNU in patients receiving NAC could not be reliably established.

The delay in RNU can be caused by a number of reasons, both disease and patient-related. In some analyzed studies longer waiting time was mainly caused by NAC and URS prior to the surgery [11,12]; however, several studies did not provide specific causes of RNU delay. Potential reasons for the delay, such as limited surgical schedules, delayed referral to urologist due to high burden on the health systems, contraindications to surgery, patients' attitude should be considered as important factors that occur in clinical practice. Delayed surgical wait times have an unfavorable impact on the overall quality of life and psychological comfort of the patients. Various studies confirmed that long waiting for surgery aggravates anxiety and psychological distress in patients with various urologic neoplasms [22,23]. The delay can also influence the patients' close relatives, increasing stress and creating frustration. What is more, the psychological well-being of patients is crucial in postoperative compliance and maintaining a positive relationship with the physicians. That is why mental health can influence the oncological outcomes in patients with UTUC and should not be underestimated.

Although the delay of a radical treatment in patients with UTUC seems to be safe and acceptable up to 3 months, it needs to be emphasized that the current data are not sufficient to reliably consider this as strong evidence. There are many potential causes of delay in RNU that could occur in clinical practice. Thus, the delay of a definitive treatment in patients with UTUC should be done with caution and rational basis in each individual case. On the basis of our synthesized data, we recommend further studies to prospectively assess the association between RNU delay and oncological outcomes in UTUC patients. Future studies should include homogenous populations in terms of causes of RNU delay (e.g., NAC administration or URS procedure before RNU) or provide detailed subgroup analyses. This could help elucidate the oncologic impact of particular delays and prepare for future unexpected events that could result in prolonged delays in definitive care in patients with UTUC.

Several limitations of the present work should be mentioned. The first and most important limitation is the retrospective and heterogeneous nature of included studies. Second, most articles did not report the reason for RNU delay. Due to possible selection bias, elderly patients with more comorbidities could be more likely to be selected for the delayed RNU than younger patients without comorbidities (possible attrition bias). Third, the studies included in our paper were conducted in different geographical regions and observed differences in the results might reflect regional ethnic differences. Fourth, as highlighted by their large CIs and small sample size, some studies might be underpowered to detect a difference in oncological outcomes between analyzed delay intervals. Fifth, the reasons of longer waiting time were not reported in some of the selected studies, thus, results of this study may not be applicable for specific subsets of patients (e.g., receiving

NAC, patients with <pT2 tumors). Finally, the planned meta-analysis was not possible because of the heterogeneity of available data.

5. Conclusions

According to the current evidence, long surgical waiting time for RNU (especially more than 3 months after UTUC diagnosis) could be considered as an important risk factor having a negative impact on oncological outcomes in patients with UTUC; however, the results of the particular studies are still inconsistent. The safe delay for RNU might be shorter in specific subsets of high-risk patients, such as those with UT and/or hydronephrosis at the time of diagnosis. Nonetheless, high-quality additional studies are required to establish evidence for valid recommendations.

Supplementary Materials: The following supporting information can be downloaded at: https://www.mdpi.com/article/10.3390/jcm11144007/s1. Figure S1. Forest plot of overall-survival data [9,12,14,15]. Short RNU delay was defined as: ≤90 days (Lee H.Y. et al. and Sundi et al.); 8–30 days (Xia et al.); ≤60 days (Zhao et al.). Long RNU delay was defined as: >90 days (Lee H.Y. et al. and Sundi et al.); 121–180 days (Xia et al.); >60 days (Zhao et al.). CI = confidence interval; IV = inverse variance; RNU = radical nephroureterectomy; SE = standard error.

Author Contributions: Conceptualization, Ł.N. and W.K.; methodology, Ł.N., J.Ł. and W.K.; software, Ł.N.; validation, W.K. and T.S.; formal analysis, W.K. and T.S.; funding acquisition, Ł.N. and B.M.; investigation, all authors; resources, all authors; data curation, Ł.N.; writing—original draft preparation, all authors; writing—review and editing, Ł.N., W.K. and P.R.; visualization, Ł.N. and W.K.; supervision, T.S. and S.F.S.; project administration, W.K. and T.S. All authors have read and agreed to the published version of the manuscript.

Funding: This research has been supported by a research grant from Wroclaw Medical University (SUBZ.C090.22.057).

Institutional Review Board Statement: Not applicable.

Informed Consent Statement: Not applicable.

Data Availability Statement: Not applicable.

Acknowledgments: The authors thank to all the members of European Association of Urology (EAU)—Young Academic Urologists (YAU) Urothelial Cancer Working Party: M. Moschini, M. Abufaraj, S. Albisinni, A. Aziz, A. Cimadamore, D. D'Andrea, W. Krajewski, E. Laukhtina, A. Mari, K. Mori, B. Pradere, F. Soria, W.S. Tan, Y.C.J. Teoh, D.M. Carrión Monsalve, E. Di Trapani, R. Flippot, A. Gallioli, J. Khalifa, G. Marcq, L.S. Mertens, R. Pichler, K.H. Tully, F. Del Giudice.

Conflicts of Interest: The authors declare no conflict of interest.

References

1. Siegel, R.L.; Miller, K.D.; Fuchs, H.E.; Jemal, A. Cancer Statistics, 2021. *CA Cancer J. Clin.* **2021**, *71*, 7–33. [CrossRef] [PubMed]
2. Rouprêt, M.; Babjuk, M.; Burger, M.; Capoun, O.; Cohen, D.; Compérat, E.M.; Cowan, N.C.; Dominguez-Escrig, J.L.; Gontero, P.; Hugh Mostafid, A.; et al. European Association of Urology Guidelines on Upper Urinary Tract Urothelial Carcinoma: 2020 Update. *Eur. Urol.* **2021**, *79*, 62–79. [CrossRef] [PubMed]
3. Ribal, M.J.; Cornford, P.; Briganti, A.; Knoll, T.; Gravas, S.; Babjuk, M.; Harding, C.; Breda, A.; Bex, A.; Rassweiler, J.J.; et al. European Association of Urology Guidelines Office Rapid Reaction Group: An Organisation-wide Collaborative Effort to Adapt the European Association of Urology Guidelines Recommendations to the Coronavirus Disease 2019 Era. *Eur. Urol.* **2020**, *78*, 21–28. [CrossRef] [PubMed]
4. Stensland, K.D.; Morgan, T.M.; Moinzadeh, A.; Lee, C.T.; Briganti, A.; Catto, J.W.F.; Canes, D. Considerations in the Triage of Urologic Surgeries During the COVID-19 Pandemic. *Eur. Urol.* **2020**, *77*, 663–666. [CrossRef] [PubMed]
5. Guerrieri, R.; Rovati, L.; Dell'Oglio, P.; Galfano, A.; Ragazzoni, L.; Aseni, P. Impact of the COVID-19 Pandemic on Urologic Oncology Surgery: Implications for Moving Forward. *J. Clin. Med.* **2021**, *11*, 171. [CrossRef]
6. Soualhi, A.; Rammant, E.; George, G.; Russell, B.; Enting, D.; Nair, R.; Van Hemelrijck, M.; Bosco, C. The incidence and prevalence of upper tract urothelial carcinoma: A systematic review. *BMC Urol.* **2021**, *21*, 110. [CrossRef]
7. Page, M.J.; McKenzie, J.E.; Bossuyt, P.M.; Boutron, I.; Hoffmann, T.C.; Mulrow, C.D.; Shamseer, L.; Tetzlaff, J.M.; Akl, E.A.; Brennan, S.E.; et al. The PRISMA 2020 statement: An updated guideline for reporting systematic reviews. *BMJ* **2021**, *372*, n71. [CrossRef]

8. Higgins, J.P.T.; Thomas, J.; Chandler, J.; Cumpston, M.; Li, T.; Page, M.J.; Welch, V.A. (Eds.) *Cochrane Handbook for Systematic Reviews of Interventions Version 6.1 (Updated September 2020)*; John Wiley & Sons: Chichester, UK, 2020; Available online: www.training.cochrane.org/handbook (accessed on 15 April 2022).
9. Lee, H.Y.; Chan, E.O.; Li, C.C.; Leung, D.; Li, W.M.; Yeh, H.C.; Chiu, P.K.; Ke, H.L.; Yee, C.H.; Wong, J.H.; et al. How to manage patients with suspected upper tract urothelial carcinoma in the pandemic of COVID-19? *Urol. Oncol.* **2021**, *39*, 733.e11–733.e16. [CrossRef]
10. Lee, J.N.; Kwon, S.Y.; Choi, G.S.; Kim, H.T.; Kim, T.H.; Kwon, T.G.; Kim, B.W. Impact of surgical wait time on oncologic outcomes in upper urinary tract urothelial carcinoma. *J. Surg. Oncol.* **2014**, *110*, 468–475. [CrossRef]
11. Nison, L.; Rouprêt, M.; Bozzini, G.; Ouzzane, A.; Audenet, F.; Pignot, G.; Ruffion, A.; Cornu, J.N.; Hurel, S.; Valeri, A.; et al. The oncologic impact of a delay between diagnosis and radical nephroureterectomy due to diagnostic ureteroscopy in upper urinary tract urothelial carcinomas: Results from a large collaborative database. *World J. Urol.* **2013**, *31*, 69–76. [CrossRef]
12. Sundi, D.; Svatek, R.S.; Margulis, V.; Wood, C.G.; Matin, S.F.; Dinney, C.P.; Kamat, A.M. Upper tract urothelial carcinoma: Impact of time to surgery. *Urol. Oncol.* **2012**, *30*, 266–272. [CrossRef] [PubMed]
13. Waldert, M.; Karakiewicz, P.I.; Raman, J.D.; Remzi, M.; Isbarn, H.; Lotan, Y.; Capitanio, U.; Bensalah, K.; Marberger, M.J.; Shariat, S.F. A delay in radical nephroureterectomy can lead to upstaging. *BJU Int.* **2010**, *105*, 812–817. [CrossRef] [PubMed]
14. Xia, L.; Taylor, B.L.; Pulido, J.E.; Guzzo, T.J. Impact of surgical waiting time on survival in patients with upper tract urothelial carcinoma: A national cancer database study. *Urol. Oncol.* **2018**, *36*, 10.e15–10.e22. [CrossRef] [PubMed]
15. Zhao, F.; Qi, N.; Zhang, C.; Xue, N.; Li, S.; Zhou, R.; Chen, Z.; Yao, R.; Zhu, H. Impact of Surgical Wait Time on Survival in Patients With Upper Urinary Tract Urothelial Carcinoma With Hydronephrosis. *Front. Oncol.* **2021**, *11*, 698594. [CrossRef] [PubMed]
16. Nowak, Ł.; Krajewski, W.; Chorbińska, J.; Kiełb, P.; Sut, M.; Moschini, M.; Teoh, J.Y.; Mori, K.; Del Giudice, F.; Laukhtina, E.; et al. The Impact of Diagnostic Ureteroscopy Prior to Radical Nephroureterectomy on Oncological Outcomes in Patients with Upper Tract Urothelial Carcinoma: A Comprehensive Systematic Review and Meta-Analysis. *J. Clin. Med.* **2021**, *10*, 4197. [CrossRef]
17. Gadzinski, A.J.; Roberts, W.W.; Faerber, G.J.; Wolf, J.S., Jr. Long-term outcomes of immediate versus delayed nephroureterectomy for upper tract urothelial carcinoma. *J. Endourol.* **2012**, *26*, 566–573. [CrossRef]
18. Gurbuz, C.; Youssef, R.F.; Shariat, S.F.; Lotan, Y.; Wood, C.G.; Sagalowsky, A.I.; Zigeuner, R.; Kikuchi, E.; Weizer, A.; Raman, J.D.; et al. The impact of previous ureteroscopic tumor ablation on oncologic outcomes after radical nephroureterectomy for upper urinary tract urothelial carcinoma. *J. Endourol.* **2011**, *25*, 775–779. [CrossRef]
19. Krajewski, W.; Nowak, Ł.; Małkiewicz, B.; Chorbińska, J.; Kiełb, P.; Poterek, A.; Sporniak, B.; Sut, M.; Moschini, M.; Lonati, C.; et al. The Impact of Primary Tumor Location on Long-Term Oncological Outcomes in Patients with Upper Tract Urothelial Carcinoma Treated with Radical Nephroureterectomy: A Systematic Review and Meta-Analysis. *J. Pers. Med.* **2021**, *11*, 1363. [CrossRef]
20. Leow, J.J.; Chong, Y.L.; Chang, S.L.; Valderrama, B.P.; Powles, T.; Bellmunt, J. Neoadjuvant and Adjuvant Chemotherapy for Upper Tract Urothelial Carcinoma: A 2020 Systematic Review and Meta-analysis, and Future Perspectives on Systemic Therapy. *Eur. Urol.* **2021**, *79*, 635–654. [CrossRef]
21. Kim, D.K.; Cho, K.S. Neoadjuvant chemotherapy for upper tract urothelial carcinoma. *Transl. Cancer Res.* **2020**, *9*, 6576–6582. [CrossRef]
22. Seklehner, S.; Hladschik-Kermer, B.; Lusuardi, L.; Schabauer, C.; Riedl, C.; Engelhardt, P.F. Psychological stress assessment of patients suffering from prostate cancer. *Scand. J. Urol.* **2013**, *47*, 101–107. [CrossRef] [PubMed]
23. Bourgade, V.; Drouin, S.J.; Yates, D.R.; Parra, J.; Bitker, M.O.; Cussenot, O.; Rouprêt, M. Impact of the length of time between diagnosis and surgical removal of urologic neoplasms on survival. *World J. Urol* **2014**, *32*, 475–479. [CrossRef] [PubMed]

MDPI
St. Alban-Anlage 66
4052 Basel
Switzerland
www.mdpi.com

Journal of Clinical Medicine Editorial Office
E-mail: jcm@mdpi.com
www.mdpi.com/journal/jcm

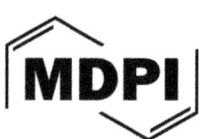

Disclaimer/Publisher's Note: The statements, opinions and data contained in all publications are solely those of the individual author(s) and contributor(s) and not of MDPI and/or the editor(s). MDPI and/or the editor(s) disclaim responsibility for any injury to people or property resulting from any ideas, methods, instructions or products referred to in the content.

www.ingramcontent.com/pod-product-compliance
Lightning Source LLC
LaVergne TN
LVHW070601100526
838202LV00012B/535